SlowItDownCKD 2019

When my family doctor told me that I probably had a problem and it had to do with my kidneys, maybe Chronic Kidney Disease, my first reaction was to demand in no uncertain terms, "What is it and how did I get it?" Hence, the title of my first CKD book.

There are many, many of us out there. By us, I mean those who have Chronic Kidney Disease. Friends and family of CKD patients can also gain some insight into the daily travails of living with the disease via this book of 2019's **SlowItDownCKD** blogs. This is not an improvement over the last books in the **SlowItDownCKD** series, but an addition which covers topics I hadn't thought of in previous years or those that readers asked about last year.

I am no expert nor am I a doctor, but I did want to know what was happening to me on a daily basis, what the medications that were ordered for me were supposed to do, and what new discoveries there were that might help slow down this deterioration of my kidneys. Apparently, so do my readers. That's what this collection of 2019's blogs is about.

The more you know about Chronic Kidney Disease, the more comfortable you'll feel in the early or moderate stages of having the disease yourself. I sure wish someone had blogged about it when it was new to me.

At one point, I discovered I had something like 17,000 readers in 106 countries and they're not afraid to tell me what they want to know. I research for them and respond with a blog post, but remind them they need to speak with their nephrologist and/or renal nutritionist before taking any action. And I repeatedly remind my readers that I am not a doctor.

I've written other books about Chronic Kidney Disease that you'll referenced many times in the blogs. Those books are ***What Is It and How Did I Get It? Early Stage Chronic Kidney Disease, SlowItDownCKD 2011, SlowItDownCKD 2012, SlowItDownCKD 2013, SlowItDownCKD 2014, SlowItDownCKD 2015, SlowItDownCKD 2016, SlowItDownCKD 2017,*** *and* ***SlowItDownCKD 2018***.

This book is extremely late in being published this year. I can only attribute that to the journey with pancreatic cancer that took most of my energy. Surprisingly, I learned quite a bit about my kidneys via this journey.

In the interest of keeping this book from becoming mammoth, I've removed the pictures, diagrams, and news of past events. I also removed my signature closing: "Until next week, keep living your life!" After all, how many times can you read the same sentence in a single book?

Welcome to ***SlowItDownCKD 2019.***

## 1/7/19 *At the Heart of the Matter*

Happy New Year! Here's wishing you all a very healthy one. I, on the other hand, found myself in the cardiologist's office the very first week of 2019. That was odd for me.

It all started when I asked my very thorough primary care physician what – if anything – it meant that my blood pressure reading was ten points higher in one arm than the other. By the way, she's the one that suggested I take my blood pressure on a daily basis. Her nurse always used the left arm to take the reading, so I did too. Then I got curious about what the reading on the other arm would be and how much difference there would be between arms. I expected a point or two, not ten.

Although my readings had always been a bit high, they weren't high enough to warrant extra attention... until I mentioned the ten point difference to my PCP. BAM! I had an appointment with the cardiologist.

This information in last year's April 23's blog will explain why:

"We know that hypertension is the number two cause of CKD. Moderating our blood pressure will (hopefully) slow down the progression of the decline of our kidney function. Kidney & Urology Foundation of America, Inc. Kidney & Urology Foundation of America, Inc. explains this succinctly:

'High blood pressure makes your heart work harder and, over time, can damage blood vessels throughout your body. If the blood vessels in your kidneys are damaged, they may stop removing wastes and extra fluid from your body. The extra fluid in your blood vessels may then raise blood pressure even more. It's a dangerous cycle.'

And heart rate? The conclusion of a study published in the Journal of Nephrology reads:

'Heart rate is an independent age-dependent effect modifier for progression to kidney failure in CKD patients.'"

So we know that blood pressure and heart rate are important for Chronic Kidney Disease patients. Just in case you've forgotten, heart rate is a synonym for pulse which is the number of times your heart beats a minute.

MedicineNet offers more about what the difference between readings from both arms MAY mean:

"People whose systolic blood pressure — the upper number in their reading — is different in their left and right arms may be suffering from a vascular disease that could increase their risk of death, British researchers report.

The arteries under the collarbone supply blood to the arms, legs and brain. Blockage can lead to stroke and other problems, the researchers noted, and measuring blood pressure in both arms should be routine.

'This is an important [finding] for the general public and for primary care doctors,' said Dr. William O'Neill, a professor of cardiology and executive dean of clinical affairs at the University of Miami Miller School Of Medicine.

'Traditionally, most people just check blood pressure in one arm, but if there is a difference, then one of the arteries has disease in it,' he said.

The arteries that run under the collarbone can get blocked, especially in smokers and diabetics, he noted. 'If one artery is more blocked than the other, then there is a difference in blood pressure in the arms,' O'Neill explained.

'Doctors should, for adults — especially adult smokers and diabetics — at some point check the blood pressure in both arms,' he said. 'If there is a difference it should be looked into further.'

The report appears in the Jan. 30 online edition of *The Lancet*."

Notice I capitalized *may*. That's because, in my case, there apparently was no blockage. My cardiologist had a different view of things. He felt there wasn't a problem unless the difference in readings between your two arms is more than 20 points and that your blood pressure would have to be much higher than my slightly elevated blood pressure before this could be considered a problem.

He made note of my diabetes and congratulated me for taking such good care of myself, especially since I'm a caretaker. I must have looked puzzled because he went on to explain that caretakers sometimes have a sort of martyr complex and are convinced they cannot take the time away from the person they're caring for to care for themselves. And, yes, he did use the oxygen masks in an airplane analogy to point out how important it is for caretakers to care for themselves first.

## 1/14/19 **And Yet Again**

I didn't think I'd be writing about the flu this year, yet I am. Why? Because, despite thinking I was safe since I didn't have it in December as usual, I have it now. Actually, I'm in the I-feel-like-an-old-dishrag stage now. Humph, that's probably why it took me six days to do the laundry (I'm still not done with the putting away) and the dishes. We were lucky enough to have my daughter and new son-in-law do the marketing for us. But it was only then that it became apparent she has it, too.

I have written before about the fact that the flu shot doesn't guarantee you won't get the flu, but that if you are one of the unlucky ones to get the flu after the shot, it will not be as virulent. Thank goodness. It's day seven and I'm just now reaching the stage where I can do something… writing, dishes, laundry…IF I get back into bed for at least an hour between tasks. To be honest, sometimes I have to interrupt those tasks to take that hour rest.

But what's different about the flu and the flu shot this year, I wondered as soon as I felt better enough to wonder about anything. This is the latest information from the Centers for Disease Control and Prevention (CDC).

"**January 11, 2019** – With the 2018-2019 flu season well underway, CDC today estimated that so far this season, between about 6 million and 7 million people have been sick with flu, up to half of those people have sought medical care for their illness, and between 69,000 and 84,000 people have been hospitalized from flu. CDC expects flu activity to continue for weeks and continues to recommend flu vaccination and appropriate use of antiviral medications.

Flu vaccination is the first line of defense to prevent flu and its potentially serious complications, including death in children. Flu vaccines have been shown to be life-saving in children, in addition to having other benefits. Flu vaccination has been shown in several studies to reduce severity of illness in people who get vaccinated but still get sick. Antiviral drugs are a second line of defense that can be used to treat flu illness. CDC recommends that people who are very sick or people who are at high risk of serious flu complications who develop flu symptoms should see a health care provider early in their illness for possible treatment with a flu antiviral drug.

CDC's weekly FluView reports when and where influenza activity is occurring, what influenza viruses are circulating and their properties, and reports the impact influenza is having on hospitalization and deaths in the United States based on data collected from eight different surveillance systems.

So far this season, H1N1 viruses have predominated nationally, however in the southeast, H3N2 viruses have been most commonly reported. The number of states reporting widespread activity increased this week to 30 from 24 states last week. While levels of influenza-like-illness (ILI) declined slightly over the previous week in this week's report, ILI remains elevated and 15 states and New York City continue to experience high flu activity. There also was a decline in the percent of respiratory specimens testing positive for flu at clinical laboratories however this number remains elevated also. During some previous seasons, drops in ILI and the percent of specimens testing positive for flu have been observed following the holidays."

Surprisingly to me, Business Insider answered my question about how the flu shot is different this year.

"The formulation has been changed in two key ways: the nasty H3N2 strain that sickened many people last year has been updated, and the influenza B virus targeted for protection in the vaccine has been changed, too. So far, the revamped vaccines look promising.

'It appears that the virus is doing a little better job, if we look at what's gone on in the southern hemisphere season,' Webby said. [Richard Webby, an infectious disease expert at St Jude Children's Research Hospital.]'

Down south in Australia, for example, it's been a fairly mild flu season, with flu activity circulating at 'low' levels, according to the Australian Department of Health. That may not perfectly translate to an equally mild flu season up north, but what Webby's seen so far suggests that the shot is also combatting the flu better than it did last year."

Okay, I took the vaccine, am having a less virulent bout of the flu but it's still here. Now what? The Kidney Foundation of Canada offered a succinct answer:

1. "For most people with kidney disease, acetaminophen (Tylenol®) is safe to use for headache, pain and fever.

2. Cold and flu medications that contain decongestants may increase blood pressure. In addition, avoid cough and cold medications that contain ASA or NSAIDs (Non-steroidal anti-inflammatory medications) such as ibuprofen (Advil®, Motrin®) or naproxen (Aleve®). If you have to use a decongestant, use a nasal spray or nasal drops. (Note: these nasal sprays are habit forming. If you use them more than three days in a row, the blood vessels in your nose can become dependent on the spray.)

3. Sore throat? Many cough syrups and throat lozenges contain sugar. Make sure you read the label to check the ingredients list, prior to use. Some sugar free or sucrose-free products are available on the market. Gargling with salt water may also be an effective way to soothe a sore throat.

4. Avoid herbal remedies. Herbal medications and products are not regulated in the same way that pharmaceutical products are. Therefore, the list of ingredients is not always accurate and some herbal medicines have been found to contain pesticides, poisonous plants, hormones, heavy metals and other compounds that are potentially dangerous. Some herbal medications also include diuretics, high levels of potassium, and/or other ingredients that can affect the kidneys or interact with your prescription medications to change their effectiveness.

5. Vitamin C is not the answer. High doses of vitamin C (500 mg or more) can cause damage to kidneys. There is a specially formulated multivitamin for people with kidney disease that has the right amount of vitamins that your kidneys can handle. Ask your healthcare team about this.

Questions? Your pharmacist and members of your kidney health team are the best source of information. Ensure you read the label, even on over the counter medications that you've taken before, as ingredients do change from time to time. If you have severe symptoms that are lasting longer than 7 days, you should see your doctor."

## 1/21/19 *Double Whammy*

Just as the flu was walking out the door, sinusitis walked in. No fair! Although, I must be feeling better because I'm starting to open all the doors and windows again.

I live in Arizona. We don't have an actual winter, but we do have a flu season with all its accompanying ailments. Having a compromised immune system is not exactly a first choice, but I have Chronic Kidney Disease.

I know I need to slow down with this explanation. Good thinking. First off, what is the immune system? I went to NCBI, The National Center for Biotechnology Information for an answer.

"The immune system (from the Latin word immunis, meaning: 'free' or 'untouched') protects the body like a guardian from harmful influences from the environment and is essential for survival. It is made up of different organs, cells and proteins and aside from the nervous system, it is the most complex system that the human body has.

As long as our body's system of defense is running smoothly, we do not notice the immune system. And yet, different groups of cells work together and form alliances against just about any pathogen (germ). But illness can occur if the performance of the immune system is compromised, if the pathogen is especially aggressive, or sometimes also if the body is confronted with a pathogen it has not come into contact before."

Notice the word "compromised" in the last sentence. According to Dictionary.com, that is

"unable to function optimally, especially with regard to immune response, owing to underlying disease, harmful environmental exposure, or the side effects of a course of treatment."

So when you have a compromised immune system, you are not receiving the full protection against germs that you could be receiving. Well, how does CKD affect the immune system?

My GFR is usually between 49% and 59%. That means at any given time I'm missing quite a bit of the function normal kidneys would have. In other words, my kidneys are working more than twice as hard as those of someone without kidney disease. This is a fact that's easy to forget now that I have the renal diet down pat … until I get sick… and it takes me longer to recuperate… or I slide right into another illness.

Let's take a look at the jobs performed by the kidneys to see exactly why. This is what I wrote in *SlowItDownCKD 2014*:

"Your kidneys filter toxins and waste products from your blood. They also regulate electrolyte levels and blood pressure and produce hormones, among their many jobs."

Let's say I eat some bad food. It would take me more than twice as long to recover and I could be more than twice as sick since my kidneys are compromised. Or maybe I actually took one of Bear's medications instead of my own (which will never happen since they're kept far, far from mine. This is just an example.) Same thing. I only have less than half the ability to remove a toxin from my body as someone with normal kidney function does. As for germs? You guessed it. My compromised immune system leaves me open to far more than I would be if I didn't have CKD.

Now for sinusitis. I had that covered in *SlowItDownCKD 2013*:

The Mayo Clinic has this to say about acute sinusitis:

'Acute sinusitis (acute rhinosinusitis) causes the cavities around your nasal passages (sinuses) to become inflamed and swollen. This interferes with drainage and causes mucus to build up.

With acute sinusitis, it may be difficult to breathe through your nose. The area around your eyes and face may feel swollen, and you may have throbbing facial pain or a headache.'

Before we get any more detailed here, a few reminders are in order {taken from **What Is It and How Did I Get It? Early Stage Chronic Kidney Disease**'s Glossary}.

Acute – Extremely painful, severe or serious, quick onset, of short duration; the opposite of chronic.

Antibiotic – Medication used to treat infection.

Chronic – Long term, the opposite of acute.

GFR – Glomerular filtration rate [if there is a lower case "e" before the term, it means estimated glomerular filtration rate] which determines both the stage of kidney disease and how well the kidneys are functioning."

Keeping it plain and simple, that just about covers my double whammy of sliding from the flu into sinusitis.

## 1/28/19 *I'll be Glowing!*

Not really, but that was my first thought when a nuclear medicine (NM) test was ordered for me. It required radioactive material to be injected into my veins. The test is called NM Hepatobiliary Scan with Pharmacologic Intervention.

Let's get a definition of hepatobiliary before we do anything else. Thank you MedicineNet for this one:

"Hepatobiliary: Having to do with the liver plus the gallbladder, bile ducts, or bile. For example, MRI (magnetic resonance imaging) can be applied to the hepatobiliary system. Hepatobiliary makes sense since 'hepato-' refers to the liver and '-biliary' refers to the gallbladder, bile ducts, or bile."

That's my kind of definition. Clear and easy for those of us who are not doctors to understand. It makes sense, too, since we were exploring what I called discomfort and my PCP called pain just under the lowest rib on my right side... very close to the gall bladder. The more than occasional nausea helped her to decide this test was necessary.

According to the test report, this is how it works:

"TECHNIQUE:

Frontal standing images of the abdomen and pelvis were obtained immediately and 30 minutes following the intravenous administration of Tc99m IDA. Pharmacologic intervention with CCK (or equivalent) and/or morphine with additional dynamic imaging was also performed."

I didn't know what Tc99mIDA or CCK was, so I'm guessing you

don't either. Wikipedia tells us,

"Technetium ($^{99m}$Tc) mebrofenin is a diagnostic radiopharmaceutical used for imaging of the liver and the gallbladder."

Hmmm, we could have figured that out from the way the term is used in the context of the technique.

Let's try CCK. This is also from Wikipedia.

"Cholecystokinin (CCK or CCK-PZ; from Greek chole, "bile"; cysto, "sac"; kinin, "move"; hence, move the bile-sac (gallbladder)) [sic] is a peptide hormone of the gastrointestinal system responsible for stimulating the digestion of fat and protein. Cholecystokinin, officially called pancreozymin, is synthesized and secreted by enteroendocrine cells in the duodenum, the first segment of the small intestine."

Well, that's fairly explanatory, but keep in mind that Wikipedia entries can be edited by anyone.

I know, now you want to know the results. Back to the test report:

"HIDA scan:

Gallbladder clearly visualized. Gallbladder ejection fraction calculated at 37% at 30 minutes. Greater than 35% is normal.

Study Result Impression:

Gallbladder clearly visualized. Borderline abnormal gallbladder response to cholecystokinin challenge."

Here's where I got lost. If my gall bladder ejection fraction is normal, how can I have a borderline abnormal gall bladder response to cholecystokinin challenge? Yep, it's time to make an appointment with my family doctor since she ordered these tests and, being who she is, can probably explain that in terms I can understand. More on that after next week's liver MRI and an appointment with her to discuss the findings of both tests.

While this is all interesting, what does it have to do with the kidneys? I went back to **SlowItDownCKD 2013** to find out what I'd written about that after my New York daughter's gall bladder was removed.

"After speaking with my daughter, I still wondered what gallstones have to do with Chronic Kidney Disease. Searching the web only garnered this one article from January, 2009 ... and the study only covered Taiwan. Of course, I found it at the National Institutes of Health.

'The prevalence of gallbladder stones in patients with Chronic Kidney Disease is significantly higher than in those without Chronic Kidney Disease. Our findings suggest that increasing age, Chronic Kidney Disease, body mass index > or =27 kg/m {greater than 59 pounds}, metabolic syndrome, and cirrhosis are the related factors for gallbladder stone formation.'

Now think about it another way: you already have a compromised immune system because you have CKD. Gallstones can cause infection of the gallbladder. As in Nima's experience, infection causes white blood cell elevation. So you know you have an infection, you might even realize it could be in the bile ducts, too. But did you check to see if there's infection in other areas of your body? That would mean you can read your own test results or have the kind of relationship with your doctors – especially your nephrologist – to freely ask questions.

As for what this organ does, this is what Medline Plus had to say.

'Your gallbladder is a pear-shaped organ under your liver. It stores bile, a fluid made by your liver to digest fat. As your stomach and intestines digest food, your gallbladder releases bile through a tube called the common bile duct. The duct connects your gallbladder and liver to your small intestine.'

Keep in mind that your liver, the largest organ in your body {The skin is actually the largest organ, but it's external.} is the other organ that filters your blood. Since your CKD has been diagnosed, your liver is already working harder. Add losing your gallbladder and you've got one very hard working – possibly overworked – liver."

Needless to say, while I was taking this in stride, especially since my kidney function is the best it's been in the over a decade since I've been diagnosed with CKD, I am now eager to have the liver MRI and get back to my primary care doctor (PCP) so she can explain what a lay person can't understand from reading the results - even with further researching.

## 2/4/19 *A Little Bit of This, A Little Bit of That*

A long time reader mentioned she had a kind of kidney disease I wasn't familiar with, so I decided to find out what I could about it. Are you aware of Uromodulin Kidney Disease?

This is what the U.S. National Library of Medicine had to say:

"Uromodulin-associated kidney disease is an inherited condition that affects the kidneys. The signs and symptoms of this condition vary, even among members of the same family.

Many individuals with uromodulin-associated kidney disease develop high blood levels of a waste product called uric acid. Normally, the kidneys remove uric acid from the blood and transfer it to urine. In this condition, the kidneys are unable to remove uric acid from the blood effectively. A buildup of uric acid can cause gout, which is a form of arthritis resulting from uric acid crystals in the joints. The signs and symptoms of gout may appear as early as a person's teens in uromodulin-associated kidney disease.

Uromodulin-associated kidney disease causes slowly progressive kidney disease, with the signs and symptoms usually beginning during the teenage years. The kidneys become less able to filter fluids and waste products from the body as this condition progresses, resulting in kidney failure. Individuals with uromodulin-associated kidney disease typically require either dialysis to remove wastes from the blood or a kidney transplant between the ages of 30 and 70. Occasionally, affected individuals are found to have small kidneys or kidney cysts (medullary cysts)."

Since this is inherited, I suspect the only way to prevent it is gene editing. I researched gene editing a bit but discovered there is quite a bit of controversy as to the legal and ethical aspects of this procedure right now. However, this doesn't mean it isn't possible.

The only other information I could find was far too technical for this lay person to understand, much less explain. Readers, do you have more information?

Something else that was new to me this week: pitaya or dragon fruit. I always buy myself a birthday present and this was mine for this year. By the way, thank you to all the readers who took the time to wish me well on my 72$^{nd}$ yesterday.

Back to pitaya. According to Healthline (Thank you again for the two awards.), pitaya is:

"Dragon fruit is a tropical fruit native to Mexico and Central America. Its taste is like a combination of a kiwi and a pear…. Dragon fruit is a low-calorie fruit that is high in fiber and provides a good amount of several vitamins and minerals…. Dragon fruit contains several antioxidants that protect your cells from damage. These include betalains, hydroxycinnamates, and flavonoids…. Animal studies suggest that dragon fruit may improve insulin resistance, liver fat, and heart health. However, the results of human studies are inconsistent…. To date, there have been two reported cases of a severe allergic reaction to dragon fruit."

I like that it contains less sugar and calories than other tropical fruits, but I didn't find the taste appealing. It was bland with just a hint of a woody aftertaste. Was it too ripe? Not ripe enough? Surprisingly, my Utah raised son-in-law loves it and jumped at the chance to finish mine.

I ran into what might have been more new information this past week when the P.A. taking my husband's blood pressure used a wrist monitor on his right wrist. I was always told an arm cuff monitor was better because the pressure was only taken through one bone, whereas there are two in the wrist. I was also told that the left arm was best because it was closer to the heart. This advice was from my PCP's nurse and that of my nephrologist. However, this P.A. insisted the wrist monitor measures atomic movement of the blood so it didn't matter whether a wrist or arm cuff were used, nor which arm was used. It didn't sound right to me.

This is from **SlowItDownCKD 2014** and may be helpful here:

"Well, what about the different kinds of blood pressure monitors? I use a wrist monitor which my PCP is simply not thrilled with. Her feeling is that I'm taking my pressure through two bones, the radius and the ulna, as opposed to only one bone, the humerus, with an arm device. There's also the finger monitor, but that could be a problem if you have thin or cold fingers.

There are manual and battery operated versions of these monitors. If you use an arm monitor, be aware that larger cuffs are available if needed. The one thing most blood pressure sites agree upon is that it's not a good idea to rely on drugstore monitors for your readings."

I have been researching for over two hours. I cannot find anything about atomic movement within the blood being measured by a blood pressure monitor of any kind. I've been to professional pages, checked studies, and even looked at advertisements. So, unless you have other information, I do believe I've been had. I just can't wait to meet this young man at the follow up appointment in two weeks when I'll ask him for resources and the monitor manufacturers' information.

On another note, I've written about KDIGO during the last two years. This is from **SlowItDownCKD 2017** and was repeated in the Sept. 17th blog in 2018.

"This stands for KIDNEY DISEASE | IMPROVING GLOBAL OUTCOMES. Their homepage states:

'**KDIGO MISSION** – Improving the care and outcomes of kidney disease patients worldwide through the development and implementation of global clinical practice guidelines.'"

So why mention it again, you ask? Well, you know how I'm always saying I'm not a doctor and neither are you, but doctors need to know what we, as kidney patients, need to say. KDIGO is now inviting patients – including those with CKD – to join their patient network. What better way to be heard as a kidney patient? I joined and I hope you will, too.

## 2/11/19 **Kidney Anxiety**

I clearly remember writing about how depression, grief, and stress affect your kidneys, but not about anxiety. As Bear's pain worsens, there's a lot of that in my house recently. I don't understand why it's taking so long for his doctors to decide upon a treatment plan for him, but while they do I am one anxious person.

I went directly to my old friend, the Mayo Clinic for a set of anxiety symptoms:

"Common anxiety signs and symptoms include:

- Feeling nervous, restless or tense
- Having a sense of impending danger, panic or doom
- Having an increased heart rate
- Breathing rapidly (hyperventilation)
- Sweating
- Trembling
- Feeling weak or tired
- Trouble concentrating or thinking about anything other than the present worry
- Having trouble sleeping
- Experiencing gastrointestinal (GI) problems
- Having difficulty controlling worry
- Having the urge to avoid things that trigger anxiety"

While I don't have all these symptoms, there are at least four or five of them I can identify with.

Wait a minute. Maybe I'm barking up the wrong tree. Is my worry about Bear's pain really causing anxiety? I popped over to MedicalNewsToday for some help in figuring out just what it is that causes anxiety.

- **Environmental factors:** Elements in the environment around an individual can increase anxiety. Stress from a personal relationship, job, school, or financial predicament can contribute greatly to anxiety disorders. Even low oxygen levels in high-altitude areas can add to anxiety symptoms.

- **Genetics:** People who have family members with an anxiety disorder are more likely to have one themselves.

- **Medical factors:** Other medical conditions can lead to an anxiety disorder, such as the side effects of medication, symptoms of a disease, or stress from a serious underlying medical condition that may not directly trigger the changes seen in anxiety disorder but might be causing significant lifestyle adjustments, pain, or restricted movement.

- **Brain chemistry:** Stressful or traumatic experiences and genetic factors can alter brain structure and function to react more vigorously to triggers that would not previously have caused anxiety. Psychologists and neurologists define many anxiety and mood disorders as disruptions to hormones and electrical signals in the brain.

- **Use of or withdrawal from an illicit substance:** The stress of day-to-day living combined with any of the above might serve as key contributors to an anxiety disorder.

There are items on this list which I hadn't considered before. Years ago, when I was teaching in an old vocational high school, a student holding one of those long, heavy, solid oak window poles to open very high windows quickly spun around to answer a question and accidentally hit me in the head with the pole. That was certainly traumatic and also one of the few times I've been hospitalized.

We've pretty much figured out that there is an undiagnosed history of anxiety in the family. I'm referring to people from past generations who faced pogroms, the Depression, and even having to give up babies for adoption since that's what was done with babies from unwed mothers in that generation. Could these folks have had anxiety disorders rather than environmental anxiety? Of course, we'll never really know since they are long gone from this earth, but it is a thought.

Lightning Bolt!!! I remember visiting my buddy and her mother in San Miguel de Allende in Mexico not long after my own mother died and being anxious. I attributed it to still being in mourning for my mother. San Miguel de Allende has an elevation of 7,000 feet. Was that one of those "low oxygen levels in high-altitude area?" I didn't know, but Laura Anderson author of the *Gunnison Country Times'* article on Acli-Mate did:

"Low landers generally aren't affected by altitude until they reach 4,500 to 5,000 feet. But after that, the affects (sic) of altitude are compounded about every 1,000 feet — so the affects (sic) of going from 6,000 feet to 7000 feet can feel the same as jumping from sea level to 4,500 feet."

What in heaven's name is this doing to my kidneys, I wondered. I was surprised to find an answer… in reverse. Rather than anxiety causing a kidney problem, it seems that fear of kidney disease can cause anxiety, or at least that's what Calm claims. Be aware that they are a business and will try to sell to you.

- **"Extra Urination** Anxiety can cause more frequent urination. When you experience anxiety, the part of your brain that controls the withholding urination slows down because anxiety requires resources to be sent to other parts of your brain. This can lead to concerns over your renal health, although nothing is wrong.

- **Lower Back Pain** Lower back pain is also very common with anxiety. Lower back pain comes from severe stress and tension, and yet it's associated with some conditions that affect the kidneys as well which can have many people worried about their kidney health.

- **Life Experiences** Anyone that suffers from anxiety and has had a friend or family member diagnosed with a terrible kidney condition is at risk for developing anxiety over the idea of poor kidneys. Anxiety can turn life experiences into very real concerns, and so kidney health concerns are one of the issues that can come up when you see it in others."

- **Urine Color** Urine color is another issue that can cause anxiety. Many people check their urine color for diseases habitually, and every once in a while the color of a person's urine may be very different than what they expect. This can create concerns that the urine color changes are due to kidney problems."

What I find interesting is that kidney disease can cause frequent urination, too. Kidney disease may also cause lower back pain. If you know any CKD patients, you know we're always checking the color of our urine to make certain we're well enough hydrated.

So it seems your fear of kidney disease may cause a symptom of kidney disease... and/or possibly diabetes. All I have to say to that is make sure you take the simple urine and blood test to determine if you do really have Chronic Kidney Disease or diabetes.

2/18/19 *Bulking Up*

While I make sure to state that I'm not a doctor, I'm not always certain my readers get that. This is why I was so glad that a reader asked me a question about her doctor's advice, prefacing her question by stating that she knows I'm not a doctor. I feel better.

Her question? It's about fiber and Chronic Kidney Disease. But first, let's find out exactly what fiber is. According to Harvard's T. H. Chan School of Public Health,

"Fiber comes in two varieties, both beneficial to health:

- Soluble fiber, which dissolves in water, can help lower glucose levels as well as help lower blood cholesterol. Foods with soluble fiber include oatmeal, nuts, beans, lentils, apples and blueberries.

- Insoluble fiber, which does not dissolve in water, can help food move through your digestive system, promoting regularity and helping prevent constipation. Foods with insoluble fibers include wheat, whole wheat bread, whole grain couscous, brown rice, legumes, carrots, cucumbers and tomatoes.

The best sources of fiber are whole grain foods, fresh fruits and vegetables, legumes, and nuts."

We all know people need fiber, but do you know why? I found the answer stated the most succinctly by Verywell Fit.

"Besides reducing the glycemic effect of meals and contributing to colon health, there is evidence that fiber may benefit us in other ways. It seems to help lower cholesterol and triglycerides, and also may help to prevent:

- Ulcers, particularly in the beginning of the small intestine (duodenal ulcers)
- Diabetes
- Heart Disease
- Cancer"

As a diabetic, I understand why I need fiber, but what about as a CKD patient? DaVita has that one covered:

"Adequate fiber in the kidney diet can be beneficial to people with chronic kidney disease (CKD) because it:

- Keeps GI (gastrointestinal) function healthy
- Adds bulk to stool to prevent constipation
- Prevents diverticulosis (pockets inside the colon)
- Helps increase water in stool for easier bowel movements
- Promotes regularity
- Prevents hemorrhoids
- Helps control blood sugar and cholesterol"

Hmmm, this is very similar to reasons why everyone – CKD or not – should pay attention to fiber. But, take a look at this list of high fiber foods from the Mayo Clinic:

| "Fruits | Serving size | Total fiber (grams)* |
|---|---|---|
| Raspberries | 1 cup | 8.0 |
| Pear | 1 medium | 5.5 |
| Apple, with skin | 1 medium | 4.5 |
| Banana | 1 medium | 3.0 |
| Orange | 1 medium | 3.0 |
| Strawberries | 1 cup | 3.0 |

| Vegetables | Serving size | Total fiber (grams)* |
|---|---|---|
| Green peas, boiled | 1 cup | 9.0 |
| Broccoli, boiled | 1 cup chopped | 5.0 |
| Turnip greens, boiled | 1 cup | 5.0 |
| Brussels sprouts, boiled | 1 cup | 4.0 |
| Potato, with skin, baked | 1 medium | 4.0 |

| | | |
|---|---|---|
| Sweet corn, boiled | 1 cup | 3.5 |
| Cauliflower, raw | 1 cup chopped | 2.0 |
| Carrot, raw | 1 medium | 1.5 |

| Grains | Serving size | Total fiber (grams)* |
|---|---|---|
| Spaghetti, whole-wheat, cooked | 1 cup | 6.0 |
| Barley, pearled, cooked | 1 cup | 6.0 |
| Bran flakes | 3/4 cup | 5.5 |
| Quinoa, cooked | 1 cup | 5.0 |
| Oat bran muffin | 1 medium | 5.0 |
| Oatmeal, instant, cooked | 1 cup | 5.0 |
| Popcorn, air-popped | 3 cups | 3.5 |
| Brown rice, cooked | 1 cup | 3.5 |
| Bread, whole-wheat | 1 slice | 2.0 |
| Bread, rye | 1 slice | 2.0 |

| Legumes, nuts and seeds | Serving size | Total fiber (grams)* |
|---|---|---|
| Split peas, boiled | 1 cup | 16.0 |
| Lentils, boiled | 1 cup | 15.5 |
| Black beans, boiled | 1 cup | 15.0 |
| Baked beans, canned | 1 cup | 10.0 |
| Chia seeds | 1 ounce | 10.0 |
| Almonds | 1 ounce (23 nuts) | 3.5 |
| Pistachios | 1 ounce (49 nuts) | 3.0 |
| Sunflower kernels | 1 ounce | 3.0 |

*Rounded to nearest 0.5 gram.

Source: USDA National Nutrient Database for Standard Reference, Legacy Release"

Looks delicious, doesn't it? So what's the problem? Well, CKD patients are restricted in their diets… and even the permissible foods are restricted as far as amounts we can eat. It all depends upon our most current lab results. Do we need less potassium?

Then we need to eat even less potassium rich food. The same is true for all the electrolytes. That means our diets may not contain enough fiber.

CKD is an inflammatory disease. Fiber can lower inflammation. So what's a CKD patient to do?

My reader was recommended supplements by her doctor. One was Solfi Green, something new to me.

I went to MIMS in the Philippines (while a new site to me, they self-describe as "Asia's one-stop resource for medical news, clinical reference and education") for the ingredients. This is what I found:

"*Ingredients:* Fructose, Mixed Fruit Powder, Mixed Vegetable Powder, Soluble Dietary Fiber, Physllium (sic) Husk, Oat Fiber, Wheat Fiber, Citric Acid, Wheat Grass, Alfalfa, Rooibos Extract, Contains Permitted Food Conditioner."

Wait a minute, Psyllium Husk? I clearly remember writing that this can cause inflammation of the gastrointestinal tract. We need to decrease, not increase, inflammation as CKD patients. I would steer clear of this.

Would my reader need to steer clear if she were a dialysis or transplant patient? Drugs.com doesn't seem to think any specific dosage reduction is necessary, but they also don't mention it can cause inflammation or that it is high in potassium. Dialysis patients, beware. If you're a transplant, you simply need to watch your labs as you would anyway. Just keep in mind psyllium husk can be both an inflammatory and laxative.

Another supplement suggested to my reader is C-lium fiber. I went directly to their now defunct website and found this warning in their FAQ:

"If you have rectal bleeding, history of intestinal blockage, difficulty swallowing, diabetes mellitus, heart disease, hypertension, kidney disease, or if you are on a low-sugar or low-sodium diet, contact your doctor before taking C-Lium Fibre."

Obviously, my reader has gone to her doctor since these two supplements were prescribed by her doctor. I have to make a confession here. When something is prescribed for me, I research it. If I don't like what I find, I speak with my doctor. If she can explain in more detail or tell me something that is not in my research which I should be aware of to make an informed decision and it's all positive, I go with the prescription. If not, well….

Of course, you have to make your own decision, just as I do. Here's hoping this has helped my reader.

2/25/19 **Pancreas + Kidneys = ?**

31 years ago, my father died of pancreatic cancer. For some reason, I remember him asking me what electrolytes were as soon as he was diagnosed. I didn't know. I do now, but I don't know if there's a connection between the pancreas and the kidneys. Of course, I mean other than the fact that they are all organs in your body.

Oh, sorry, I didn't give you the definition. This is from Healthline:

" 'Electrolyte' is the umbrella term for particles that carry a positive or negative electric charge ….

In nutrition, the term refers to essential minerals found in your blood, sweat and urine.

When these minerals dissolve in a fluid, they form electrolytes — positive or negative ions used in metabolic processes.

Electrolytes found in your body include:

- Sodium
- Potassium
- Chloride
- Calcium
- Magnesium
- Phosphate
- Bicarbonate

These electrolytes are required for various bodily processes, including proper nerve and muscle function, maintaining acid-base balance and keeping you hydrated."

Ummm, you have Chronic Kidney Disease. These are the electrolytes you need to keep an eye on, especially sodium, potassium, and phosphate. But why did Dad ask me about them?

I plunged right in to find the answer and immediately found a journal article… on a pay site. Not being one to pay for what can be found for free (and is 30 years old, by the way), I decided to look for as much information on the pancreas as I could find and see what we could figure out together.

Let's start at the beginning. According to the Sol Goldman Pancreatic Cancer Research Center of Johns Hopkins Medicine – Pathology:

**"What is the pancreas?**

The pancreas is a long flattened gland located deep in the belly (abdomen). Because the pancreas isn't seen or felt in our day to day lives, most people don't know as much about the pancreas as they do about other parts of their bodies. The pancreas is, however, a vital part of the digestive system and a critical controller of blood sugar levels.

**Where is the pancreas?**

The pancreas is located deep in the abdomen. Part of the pancreas is sandwiched between the stomach and the spine. The other part is nestled in the curve of the duodenum (first part of the small intestine). To visualize the position of the pancreas, try this:

touch your right thumb and right 'pinkie' fingers together, keeping the other three fingers together and straight. Then, place your hand in the center of your belly just below your lower ribs with your fingers pointing to your left. Your hand will be the approximate shape and at the approximate level of your pancreas."

I tried that. It's not as easy as it sounds.

So now we sort of know what and where it is, but what does it do? No problem, Columbia University Irving Medical Center has just the info we need:

**"Exocrine Function:**

The pancreas contains exocrine glands that produce enzymes important to digestion. These enzymes include trypsin and chymotrypsin to digest proteins; amylase for the digestion of carbohydrates; and lipase to break down fats. When food enters the stomach, these pancreatic juices are released into a system of ducts that culminate in the main pancreatic duct. The pancreatic duct joins the common bile duct to form the ampulla of Vater which is located at the first portion of the small intestine, called the duodenum. The common bile duct originates in the liver and the gallbladder and produces another important digestive juice called bile. The pancreatic juices and bile that are released into the duodenum help the body to digest fats, carbohydrates, and proteins.

**Endocrine Function:**

The endocrine component of the pancreas consists of islet cells (islets of Langerhans) that create and release important hormones directly into the bloodstream. Two of the main pancreatic hormones are insulin, which acts to lower blood sugar, and glucagon, which acts to raise blood sugar. Maintaining proper blood sugar levels is crucial to the functioning of key organs including the brain, liver, and kidneys."

The kidneys? Now it's starting to make sense. We need whatever specific electrolyte balance our lab work tells us we need to keep our kidneys working in good stead and we need a well-functioning pancreas to regulate our blood sugars. Hmmm, diabetes is one of the two leading causes of CKD. It seems the pancreas controls diabetes since it creates insulin.

What could happen if the pancreas wasn't doing its job, I wondered. This is from the Mayo Clinic,

"Pancreatitis [Me here: that's an inflammation of the pancreas] can cause serious complications, including:

- **Pseudocyst.** Acute pancreatitis can cause fluid and debris to collect in cystlike pockets in your pancreas. A large pseudocyst that ruptures can cause complications such as internal bleeding and infection.

- **Infection.** Acute pancreatitis can make your pancreas vulnerable to bacteria and infection. Pancreatic infections are serious and require intensive treatment, such as surgery to remove the infected tissue.

- **Kidney failure.** Acute pancreatitis may cause kidney failure, which can be treated with dialysis if the kidney failure is severe and persistent.

- **Breathing problems.** Acute pancreatitis can cause chemical changes in your body that affect your lung function,

- causing the level of oxygen in your blood to fall to dangerously low levels.

- **Diabetes.** Damage to insulin-producing cells in your pancreas from chronic pancreatitis can lead to diabetes, a disease that affects the way your body uses blood sugar.

- **Malnutrition.** Both acute and chronic pancreatitis can cause your pancreas to produce fewer of the enzymes that are needed to break down and process nutrients from the food you eat. This can lead to malnutrition, diarrhea and weight loss, even though you may be eating the same foods or the same amount of food.

- **Pancreatic cancer.** Long-standing inflammation in your pancreas caused by chronic pancreatitis is a risk factor for developing pancreatic cancer.

Did you catch kidney failure and diabetes? I believe we now know how the kidneys and pancreas are related to each other. Ah, if only I'd known how to research 31 years ago….

## 3/4/19 *National Kidney Month, 2019*

Anyone remember LOL? It's older internet shorthand for Laughing Out Loud. That's what I'm doing right now. Why? Because, after all these years of blogging, I've just realized that I compose my opening paragraph as I'm waking up. Still in bed, mind you. Still half asleep. Isn't the brain wonderful?

This is my half asleep composition for this morning: March is National Kidney Month. That's not to be confused with March 14$^{th}$, which is World Kidney Day. So, today, we address the nation. Next week, the world.

As usual, let's start at the beginning. What is National Kidney Month? Personalized Cause has a succinct explanation for us. By the way, while I'm not endorsing them since the site is new to me, I should let you know they sell the green ribbons for National Kidney Month that you'll probably be seeing hither and yon all month.

"National Kidney Month, observed in March and sponsored by the *National Kidney Foundation*, is a time to increase awareness of kidney disease, promote the need for a cure, and spur advocacy on behalf of those suffeing (sic) with the emotional, financial and physical burden of kidney disease. The *National Kidney Foundation* is the leading organization in the U.S. dedicated to the awareness, prevention and treatment of kidney disease for hundreds of thousands of healthcare professionals, millions of patients and their families, and tens of millions of Americans at risk."

That, of course, prompted me to go directly to the National Kidney Foundation's information about National Kidney Month.

"Focus on the Kidneys During National Kidney Month in March

March is National Kidney Month and the NKF is urging all Americans to give their kidneys a second thought and a well-deserved checkup. Kidneys filter 200 liters of blood a day, help regulate blood pressure and direct red blood cell production. But they are also prone to disease; 1 in 3 Americans is at risk for kidney disease due to diabetes, high blood pressure or a family history of kidney failure. There are more than 30 million Americans who already have kidney disease, and most don't know it because there are often no symptoms until the disease has progressed."

This is also the month of kidney walks, like the one my daughter Nima participated in on the East Coast in my honor, or the one for which I organized a team several years ago. Actually, it's the month specifically for anything and everything that will raise awareness of kidney disease. I've mentioned that I contributed a chapter to the book *1in9*, which is about kidney disease. You're right. The book launch is this month….

The American Kidney Fund is also taking part in National Kidney Month. I wanted to share this quote from the AKF with you, both as a CKD awareness advocate and a woman:

"'Kidney disease is a silent killer that disproportionately affects women who are often the primary caregivers for loved ones with the disease, are more likely to become living donors but less likely to receive a transplant, and are at higher risk for CKD,' said LaVarne A. Burton, president and chief executive officer of AKF. 'Because women with kidney disease may also face other health issues, including infertility, pregnancy complications, bone disease and depression, AKF is using Kidney Month to let women know we are here to support them and to provide resources that will answer their questions and concerns.'"

The Renal Support Network is working even more emphatically to spread kidney disease awareness this month, too:

"March is National Kidney Month. This is a special time set aside to raise awareness about kidney health and activities. RSN invites members of the kidney community, our friends and our families to join in the conversation."

This on top of their usual. For those that are not familiar with this group, the following statement is from their website.

"Since 1993 RSN has created and continues to produce a vast collection of information about kidney disease. Feel free to share our National Kidney Month page, a favorite story, KidneyTalk™ show or awareness image on social media using the hashtag #KidneyMonth and be sure to tag us @RSNhope."

DaVita Kidney Care offers many resources (as the website's title assures us) to help understand both CKD and dialysis. Some of their offerings are:

- "Organizations and Programs
- Education
- Advice & Inspiration
- Recipes & Nutrition
- Specific Kidney Diseases
- Resources
- Health Related Portals"

As for me, I'll blog my brains out until more and more people are aware of kidney disease. Same goes for the Instagram, Facebook, Twitter, Pinterest, and LinkedIn accounts. It's all about kidney disease.

### 3/11/19 *World Kidney Day, 2019*

Will you look at that? The world keeps moving on no matter what's going on in our personal lives. And so, I recognize that Thursday of this week is World Kidney Day. In honor of this occasion, I've chosen to update last year's World Kidney Day blog... so sit back and enjoy the read.

...World Kidney Day? What's that? I discovered this is a fairly new designation. It was only thirteen years ago that it was initiated.

According to worldkidneyday.org,

"World Kidney Day is a global awareness campaign aimed at raising awareness of the importance of our kidneys."

Sound familiar? That's where I'm heading with ***What Is It and How Did I Get It? Early Stage Chronic Kidney Disease***; ***SlowItDownCKD 2011; SlowItDownCKD 2012; SlowItDownCKD 2013; SlowItDownCKD 2014; SlowItDownCKD 2015; SlowItDownCKD 2016; SlowItDownCKD 2017;*** (and now ***SlowItDownCKD 2018***) Facebook; Instagram; LinkedIn; Pinterest; Twitter; and this blog. We may be running along different tracks, but we're headed in the same direction.

The 59 year old International Society of Nephrology (ISN) – a non-profit group spreading over 155 countries – is one part of the equation for their success. Another is the International Federation of Kidney Foundations with membership in over 40 countries. Add a steering committee and The World Kidney Day Team and you have the makings of this particular concept....

According to their website (which requires login):

"The mission of World Kidney Day is to raise awareness of the importance of our kidneys to our overall health and to reduce the frequency and impact of kidney disease and its associated health problems worldwide.

Objectives:

- Raise awareness about our 'amazing kidneys'
- Highlight that diabetes and high blood pressure are key risk factors for Chronic Kidney Disease (CKD)
- Encourage systematic screening of all patients with diabetes and hypertension for CKD
- Encourage preventive behaviors
- Educate all medical professionals about their key role in detecting and reducing the risk of CKD, particularly in high risk populations
- Stress the important role of local and national health authorities in controlling the CKD epidemic."

While there are numerous objectives for this year's World Kidney Day, the one that lays closest to my heart is this one: 'Encourage systematic screening of all patients with diabetes and hypertension for CKD.'

Back to World Kidney Day's website now, if you please.

This year's theme is Kidney Health for Everyone Everywhere.

Their site offers materials and ideas for events as well as a map of global events. Prepare to be awed at how wide spread World Kidney Day events are.

Before you leave their page, take a detour to Kidney FAQ (Frequently Asked Questions) on the toolbar at the top of the page. You can learn everything you need to know from what the kidneys do to what the symptoms (or lack thereof) of CKD are, from how to treat CKD to a toolbox full of helpful education about your kidneys to preventative measures.

If only my nurse practitioner had been aware of National Kidney Month or World Kidney Day, she could have warned me immediately that I needed to make lifestyle changes so the decline of my kidney function could have been slowed down earlier. How much more of my kidney function would I still have if I'd known earlier? That was a dozen years ago. This shouldn't still be happening… but it is.

I received a phone call a few years ago that just about broke my heart. Someone very dear to me sobbed, "He's dying." When I calmed her down, she explained a parent was sent to a nephrologist who told him he has end stage renal disease and needed dialysis or transplantation immediately.

I pried a little trying to get her to admit he'd been diagnosed before end stage, but she simply didn't know what I was talking about. There had been no diagnose of Chronic Kidney Disease up to this point. There was diabetes, apparently out of control diabetes, but no one impressed upon this man that diabetes is the foremost cause of CKD.

What a waste of the precious time he could have had to do more than stop smoking, which he did (to his credit), the moment he was told it would help with the diabetes. Would he be where he was then if his medical practitioners had been aware of National Kidney Month or World Kidney Day, especially since this man was high risk due to his age and diabetes?

I have a close friend who was involved in the local senior center where she lives. She said she didn't know anyone else but me who had this disease. Since 1 out of every 7 people does nationally (That's 15% of the adult population) and being over 60 places you in a high risk group, I wonder how many of her friends were included in the 96% of those in the early stage of CKD who don't know they have CKD or don't even know they need to be tested. I'd have rather been mistaken here, but I'm afraid I wasn't. National Kidney Month or World Kidney Day could have helped them become aware.

For those of you who have forgotten (Easily read explanations of what results of the different items on your tests mean are in ***What Is It And How Did I Get It? Early Stage Chronic Kidney Disease.***), all it takes is a blood test and a urine test to detect CKD. I have routine blood tests every three months to monitor a medication I'm taking. It was in this test, a test I took anyway, that my family physician uncovered Chronic Kidney Disease as a problem.

There is so much free education about CKD online.... None of us needs to hear another sorrowful, "If only I had known!"

3/18/19 *From a Book...*

I was trying to figure out a new angle from which to write about Chronic Kidney Disease during National Kidney Month and decided that my chapter in the newly released ***1in9*** just might be the way.

By the way, I really don't like shopping, but did so for a 'fancy blouse' for the fancy book launch. The day of the launch turned out to be the day I unexpectedly had anesthesia and I ended up not being able to go. From the pictures I've seen of the event, it was a fun event. Now I need another fun event to wear that 'fancy blouse' to. After all, we can't let a dreaded shopping trip go to waste, can we?

Without further ado, I present the first part of my ***1in9*** chapter:

My name is Gail Rae-Garwood. I like to think of myself as an average older woman with two adult daughters, a fairly recent husband, and a very protective dog. But I'm not. What makes me a little different is that I have Chronic Kidney Disease… just like the estimated 30 million or 15% of the adult population in the United States. Unlike 96% of those in the early stages of the disease, I know my kidneys are not functioning well.

Once upon a time, a long, long time ago, before I'd ever heard the word nephrology, I paid no attention to my kidneys. I had just a vague idea of where they were located because I had big brothers. Every time they watched boxing, one or the other of them would yell, "Oh! Right in the kidneys!" when one guy hit the other on the back, sort of near the waist. My mother attempted to feed us kidney beans once or twice, but three voices chorusing the 1950's equivalent of "Uh, gross!" was enough to convince her they weren't that necessary. My father had a friend who'd moved up in the world and had a kidney shaped pool. Of course, I never had a bird's eye view of that as a child. So, we were a family pretty much ignorant about kidneys.

When I grew up, I never let my children watch boxing; it was too violent. I never even tried to feed them kidney beans, probably due to some residual abhorrence left over from my own childhood. I had no friends with kidney shaped pools, but I had flown in an airplane and could recognize one if we were flying low. That was the sum total of my kidney education. I didn't even recall if they were covered in high school biology. My daughters, now grown women, said they were, but I didn't remember anything about that.

I was blindsided over a decade ago. That's when I started seeing a new doctor solely because she was both on my insurance plan and so much closer to home than the one I'd been seeing. It seems everything is at least half an hour away in Arizona; her office wasn't. As a diligent primary care physician, she ordered a whole battery of tests to verify what she found in my files which, by the way, contained a kidney function reading (called the GFR) of 39%. That was something I'd never been told about.

39%. I'd been a high school teacher for 35 years at that point. If a student had scored 39% on a test, we would have talked and talked until we had gotten to the root of the problem that caused such a low score. No one talked to me about my low kidney function until I changed doctors.

"That's not normal," said my new doctor as she looked at my blood test results.

I made the supreme effort of tearing my eyes away from the height and weight chart to ask, "What's not normal?"

"Your GFR," she told me. I looked at her blankly. (In retrospect, I can understand how hard it probably was for her not to laugh at my empty eyes and a face without a shred of interest showing on it.) I said nothing. She said nothing.

Finally, I asked, "What's that?" She gave me a simple explanation with no indication that I should panic in any way, but of course I did.

"It's what! It's below normal? My kidneys aren't functioning to full capacity? Why wasn't I told? What do I do now? How do I fix the problem? I want them at 100%."

Her voice rose over mine in a steady, sure manner. "This does not mean there is a problem. It means you must go to a specialist to see if there really is a problem."

"Oh." I didn't believe her, but she not only talked, she had me in a nephrologist's (kidney and hypertension specialist) office the next day. That's when I started worrying. Who gets an appointment with a specialist the very next day? I was diagnosed at stage 3; there are only 5 stages. I had to start working to slow down the progression in the decline of my kidney function immediately.

I read just about every book I could find concerning this problem. Surprisingly, very few books dealt with the early or moderate stages of the disease. Yet these are the stages when CKD patients are most shocked, confused, and maybe even depressed—and the stages at which they have a workable chance of doing something to slow down the progression in the decline of their kidney function.

This first nephrologist might have been reassuring, but I'll never know. I was terrified; he was patriarchal. All I heard was, "I'll take care of your kidneys. You just do as I say," or something to that effect.

Nope, wrong doctor for me. I wanted to know how medication, diet, exercise and other lifestyle changes could help. I didn't want to be told what to do without an explanation as to why… and when I couldn't get an explanation that was acceptable to me, I started researching. (More about that later.) You see, I'd already had a terrific Dad who'd known better than to ask me to give up control of myself. I didn't need a doctor assuming his role… especially in a way I resented.

… to be continued. (This will take several weeks. It is a chapter in book, so it's longer than my usual 1,000 or so word blog.)

3/25/19 **To Continue…**

National Kidney Month is just flying by. This is actually the last week and I doubt I'll be able to post the rest of the **1in9** chapter before next month. But then again, it's always Kidney Month for those of us with Chronic Kidney Disease. By the way, thank you to the reader who made it a point of telling me she can't wait to read the rest of the chapter. Sooooo, let's get started!

\*\*\*

Nephrologist switch. The new one was much better for me. He explained again and again until I understood and he put up with a lot of verbal abuse when this panicky new patient wasn't getting answers as quickly as she wanted them. Luckily for me, he graciously accepted my apology.

After talking to the nephrologist, I began to realize just how serious this disease was and started to wonder why my previous nurse practitioner had not caught this. When I asked her why, she responded, "It was inconclusive testing." Sure it was. Because she never ordered the GFR tested; that had been incidental! I feel there's no sense crying over spilled milk (or destroyed nephrons, in this case), but I wonder how much more of my kidney function I could have preserved if I'd known about my CKD earlier.

According to the Mayo Clinic, there are 13 early signs of chronic kidney disease. I never experienced any of them, not even one. While I did have high blood pressure, it wasn't uncontrollable which is one of the early signs. Many, like me, never experienced any noticeable symptoms. Unfortunately, many, like me, may have had high blood pressure (hypertension) for years before CKD was diagnosed. Yet, high blood pressure and diabetes are the two leading causes of CKD. I find it confusing that uncontrollable high blood pressure may be an early sign of CKD, but hypertension itself is the second leading cause of CKD.

Here's the part about my researching. I was so mystified about what was happening and why it was happening that I began an extensive course of research. My nephrologists did explain what everything meant (I think), but I was still too shocked to understand what they were saying. I researched diagnoses, descriptions of tests, test results, doctors' reports, you name it. Slowly, it began to make sense, but that understanding only led to more questions and more research.

You've probably already guessed that my world changed during that first appointment. I began to excuse myself for rest periods each day when I went back East for a slew of family affairs right after. I counted food groups and calories at these celebrations that summer. And I used all the errand running associated with them as an excuse to speed walk wherever I went and back so I could fit in my exercise. Ah, but that was just the beginning.

My high blood pressure had been controlled for 20 years at that time, but what about my diet? I had no clue there was such a thing as a kidney diet until the nutritionist explained it to me. I'm a miller's granddaughter and ate anything – and I do mean anything - with grain in it: breads, muffins, cakes, croissants, all of it. I also liked lots of chicken and fish... not the five ounces per day I'm limited to now.

The nutritionist explained to me how hard protein is on the kidneys... as is phosphorous... and potassium... and, of course, sodium. Out went my daily banana—too high in potassium. Out went restaurant burgers—larger than my daily allowance of protein.

Chinese food? Pizza? Too high in sodium. I embraced an entirely new way of eating because it was one of the keys to keeping my kidneys functioning in stage 3.

I was in a new food world. I'd already known about restricting sodium because I had high blood pressure, but these other things? I had to keep a list of which foods contain them, how much was in each of these foods, and a running list of how much of each I had during the day so I knew when I reached my limit for that day.

Another critical piece of slowing down CKD is medication. I was already taking meds to lower my blood pressure when I was first diagnosed with CKD. Two more prescriptions have been added to this in the last decade: a diuretic that lowers my body's absorption of salt to help prevent fluid from building up in my body (edema), and a drug that widens the blood vessels by relaxing them. I take another drug for my brand new diabetes. (Bye-bye, sugars and most carbs.) The funny thing is now my favorite food is salad with extra virgin olive oil and balsamic vinegar. I never thought that would happen: I was a chocoholic!

Exercise, something I loved until my arthritis got in the way, was also important. I was a dancer. Wasn't that enough? Uh-uh, I had to learn about cardio and strength training exercise, too. It was no longer acceptable to be pleasantly plump. My kidneys didn't need the extra work. Hello to weights, walking, and a stationary bike. I think I took sleep for granted before CKD, too, and I now make it a point to get a good night's sleep. A sleep apnea device improved my sleep—and my kidney function rose.

I realized I needed to rest, too. Instead of giving a lecture, running to an audition, and coming home to meet a deadline, I slowly started easing off until I didn't feel like I was running on empty all the time. The result was that I ended up graciously retiring from both acting and teaching at a local college, which gave me more time to work on my CKD awareness advocacy.

\*\*\*

There's so much more to tell you about my personal CKD journey... and you'll read more of it next week. Although, I should remind you that the entire book is available in print and digital on both Amazon.com and B&N.com, just as the entire **SlowItDownCKD** series of books is.

4/1/19  *National Kidney Month Extended*

The chapter I contributed to *1in9* goes on beyond National Kidney Month, so since I think *every day* should be World Kidney Day, I decided to just keep printing it until it was finished. Gotcha! Bet you thought I was going to write every month should be National Kidney Month. Although, that's not a bad idea either. So, for those of you just tuning in, this is actually part three of that chapter. You can just turn back a few pages to read the first two parts. Ready? Let's go.

***

But, I had to be oh-so-vigilant with other medical practitioners. One summer I had four different infections and had to quickly research the medications prescribed in the emergency room. One hospital insisted I could take sulfa drugs because I was only stage 2 at the time. My nephrologist disagreed. They also prescribed a pain killer with acetaminophen in it, another no-no for us. I didn't return to them when I developed the other infections.

My experience demonstrates that you can slow down CKD. I was diagnosed at stage 3 and I am still there, over a decade later. It takes knowledge, commitment and discipline—but it can be done, and it's worth the effort. I'm sneaking up on 72 now and know this is where I want to spend my energy for the rest of my life: chronic kidney disease awareness advocacy. I think it's just that important.

At the time of my diagnosis, I was a college instructor. My favorite course to teach was Research Writing. I was also an author with an Academic Certificate in Creative Non-Fiction and a bunch of publications under my belt. It occurred to me that I couldn't be the only one who had no clue what this new-to-me disease was and how to handle living with it. I knew how to research and I knew how to write, so why not share what I learned?

I wasn't sure of what had to be done to share or how to do it. I learned by trial and error. People were so kind in teaching me, pointing out what might work better, even suggesting others that might be interested in what I was doing. I love people. I'd written quite a few how to(s), study guides, articles, and literary guides so the writing was not new to me. I asked for suggestions as to what to do with my writing and that's when I learned about unscrupulous, price gouging vanity publishers. I'm still paying for the unwitting mistakes I made, but they were learning experiences.

My less-than-stellar experience with being diagnosed and the first nephrologist is what prompted me to write **What Is It and How Did I Get It? Early Stage Chronic Kidney Disease.** Why, I wondered, should any new CKD patient be as terrified as I was? Of course, I constantly remind my readers that I'm not a doctor and they need to consult their nephrologists or renal dietitians before making any changes to their regiment.

I didn't feel… well, done with sharing or researching once I finished the book so I began writing a weekly blog: **SlowItDownCKD**. Well, that and because a nephrologist in India told me he wanted his newly diagnosed patients to read my book, but most of them couldn't afford the bus fare to the clinic, much less a book. I published each chapter as a blog post. The nephrologist translated my posts, printed them and distributed them to his patients—who took the printed copies back to their communities. It would work!

But first I had to teach myself how to blog. I made some boo-boos and lost a bunch of blogs until I got it figured out. So why do I keep blogging? There always seems to be more to share about CKD. Each week, I wonder what I'll write... and the ideas keep coming. I now have readers in something like 106 different countries who ask me questions I hadn't even thought of. I research for them and respond with a blog post, reminding them to speak with their nephrologists and/or renal nutritionists before taking any action... and that I'm not a doctor. The blog has won several awards. Basically, that's because I write in a reader friendly manner. After all, what good is all my researching if no one understands what I'm writing?

Non-tech savvy readers asked if I could print the blogs; hence, the birth of the **SlowItDownCKD** series of books. Some people think **SlowItDownCKD** is a business; it's not. Some think it's a profit maker; it's not. So, what is it you ask? It's a vehicle for spreading awareness of Chronic Kidney Disease and whatever goes along with the disease. Why do I do it? Because I had no idea what it was, nor how I might have prevented the disease, nor how to deal with it effectively once I was diagnosed. I couldn't stand the thought of others being in the same position.

One of my daughters taught me about social media. What???? You could post whatever you wanted to? And Facebook wasn't the only way to reach the public at large? Hello, LinkedIn. A friend who is a professional photographer asked me why I wasn't using my fun photography habit to promote awareness. What??? You could do that? Enter Instagram. My step-daughters love Pinterest. That got me to thinking and suddenly **SlowItDownCKD** had a Pinterest account. Then someone I met at a conference casually mentioned she offers Twitter workshops. What kind of workshops? She showed me how to use Twitter to raise CKD awareness.

\*\*\*

There's more and you'll get to read it next week. I hope you're enjoying your look into how I entered the world of Chronic Kidney Disease Awareness Advocacy.

*4/8/19 I'm Finally Ready to Let National Kidney Month Go*

As you already know, I've been posting the chapter I contributed to the book *1in9* as my contribution to National Kidney Month. This will probably be the final post of that chapter, unless I decide to post the biography that goes along with the chapter at a later date.

Most of you are aware that I now have pancreatic cancer and the chemo effects are getting in my way. I'm hoping that I'll not be feeling them so severely in the near future and will be able to research some new material for you. Right now, that's just not possible. You may have noticed that my Twitter, Instagram, and Facebook pages no longer contain original posts. That's due to the same reason.

But let's complete the book chapter:

When I was diagnosed back in 2008, there weren't that many reader friendly books on anything having to do with CKD. Since then, more and more books of this type have been published. I'm laughing along with you, but I don't mean just **SlowItDownCKD 2011, SlowItDownCKD 2012** (These two were **The Book of Blogs: Moderate Stage Chronic Kidney Disease, Part 1,** until I realized how unwieldy both the book and the title were – another learning experience), **SlowItDownCKD 2013, SlowItDownCKD 2014** (These two were formerly **The Book of Blogs: Moderate Stage Chronic Kidney Disease, Part 2), SlowItDownCKD 2015, SlowItDownCKD 2016,** and **SlowItDownCKD 2017.** By the way, I'm already working on **SlowItDownCKD 2018**. (Gail here: Already published and available on Amazon.com.) Each book contains the blogs for that year.

I include guest blogs or book review blogs to get a taste of the currently available CKD news. For example, **1in9** guest blogged this year. Books such as Dr. Mandip S. Kang's, **The Doctor's Kidney Diets** (which also contains so much non-dietary information that we - as CKD patients - need to know), and Drs. Raymond R. Townsend and Debbie L. Cohen's **100 Questions & Answers about Kidney Disease and Hypertension**.

I miss my New York daughter and she misses me, so we sometimes have coffee together separately. She has a cup of coffee and I do at the same time. It's not like being together in person, but it's something. You can find support the same way via Facebook Chronic Kidney Disease Support Groups. Some of these groups are:

Chronic Kidney Disease Awareness

CKD (Kidney Failure) Support Group International

Dialysis & Kidney Disease

Friends Sharing Positive Chronic Kidney Disease

I Hate Dialysis

Kidney Disease Diet Ideas and Help

Kidney Disease Ideas and Diets 1

Kidney Disease, Dialysis, and Transplant

Kidney Warriors Foundation

Kidneys and Vets

Mani Trust

Mark's Private Kidney Disease Group

P2P

People on Dialysis

Sharing a Positive Kidney Warrior Journey Together

The Transplant Community Outreach

Women's Renal Failure

What I hit over and over again in the blogs is that diabetes is the foremost cause of CKD with hypertension as the second most common cause. Simple blood and urine tests can uncover your CKD – if you're part of the unlucky 96% of those in the early stages of the disease who don't know they have it.

Each time I research, I'm newly amazed at how much there is to learn about CKD...and how many tools you have at your disposal to help slow it down. Diet is the obvious one. But if you smoke or drink, stop, or at least cut down. If you don't exercise, start. Adequate, good quality sleep is another tool. Don't underestimate rest either; you're not being lazy when you rest, you're preserving whatever kidney function you have left. I am not particularly a pill person, but if there's a medication prescribed that will slow down the gradual decline of my kidney function, I'm all for it.

I was surprised to discover that writing my **SlowItDownCKD** book series, maintaining a blog, Facebook page, Twitter, Instagram, and Pinterest accounts of the same name are not enough for me for me to spread the word about CKD screening and education. I'm determined to change this since I feel so strongly that NO ONE should have this disease and not be aware of it.

That's why I've brought CKD awareness to every community that would have me: coffee shops, Kiwanis Clubs, independent bookstores, senior citizen centers, guest blogging for the likes of The American Kidney Fund and The National Kidney Foundation, being interviewed by publications like the *Wall Street Journal*'s Health Matters, The Center for Science in The Public Interest, and The United Federation of Teachers' New York Teacher, and on podcasts such as The Renal Diet Headquarters, Online with Andrea, The Edge Podcast, Working with Chronic Illness, and Improve Your Kidney Health.

I've been very serious about sharing about CKD before it advances to end stage... meaning dialysis. To that end, I gathered a team for the National Kidney Foundation of Arizona Kidney Walk one year. Another year, I organized several meetings at the Salt River Pima-Maricopa Indian Community. Education is vital since so many people are unaware they even have the disease.

You can slow down the progression of the decline of kidney function. I have been spending a lot of time on my health and I'm happy to say it's been paying off. There are five stages. I've stayed at the middle one for over a decade despite having both high blood pressure and diabetes. That's what this is about. People don't know about CKD. They get diagnosed. They think they're going to die. Everybody dies, but it doesn't have to be of CKD. I am downright passionate about people knowing this.

Thanks for taking the time to finish the chapter. The more people who know about Chronic Kidney Disease, the more people can tell others about it. I'd hate for anyone to be part of the 96% of those with CKD who don't know they have it.

## 4/15/19 *CKD and Me*

Okay, so I was finally ready to give up World Kidney Day and National Kidney Month. Maybe it's time to give up the *1in9* chapter contribution, too. Since each contributing author also had their biography accompanying their chapter, I think the best way to do that is to print the biography… although it's all me, me, me. Indulge me, please.

\*\*\*

Ms. Rae-Garwood's writing started out as a means to an end for a single parent with two children and a need for more income than her career as a NYC teacher afforded. Gail retired from both college teaching and acting – after a bit of soul searching about where her CKD limited energy would be best spent – early in 2013. Since her diagnose, Ms. Rae-Garwood writes most often about Chronic Kidney Disease, although she does write fiction. She has a three time award winning weekly blog (Surprise!) about this topic at https://gailraegarwood.wordpress.com and social media accounts as @SlowItDownCKD.

\*\*\*

Hmmm, it seems to me I've done a lot more with Chronic Kidney Disease awareness advocacy since I started with this in 2010. Let's see what else there is. Aha! These are on my website at www.gail-raegarwood.com.

Arizona Health & Living (West Valley)   6/2018

MyTherapy Guest Blog    3/8/18

eCareDiary: Coping with Chronic Kidney Disease  3/06/18

NephJC: One More Patient Voice on CKD Staging and Precision Medicine   12/08/16

Center for Science in the Public Interest: Nutrition Action Healthletter   9/16

New York State United Teachers: It's What We Do   8/9/16

American Kidney Fund: Slowing Down CKD – It Can Be Done   7/14/16

The Edge Podcast   5/19/16

Dear Annie   3/10/14

Renal Diet Headquarters Podcast   2/12/14

Accountable Kidney Care Collaborative: Bob's Blog   1/23/14

Wall Street Journal: Patients Can Do More to Control Chronic Conditions   1/13/14

The Neuropathy Doctor's News   9/23/13

Series of five Monthly CKD education classes in The Salt River Pima-Maricopa Indian Community   9/12/13

KidneySteps: Gail Rae and *SlowItDown*   9/11/13

Salt River Pima-Maricopa Indian Community: 4th Annual Men and Women's Gathering   8/29/13

National Kidney Foundation: Staying Healthy   6/6/13

KidneySteps: Learning Helps with CKD   7/04/12

Life Options Links for Patients and Professionals   5/30/12

It Is Just What It Is   3/9/12

Online with Andrea   03/07/12

Working with Chronic Illness   2/17/12

Libre Tweet Chat with Gail Rae   1/10/12

Kevinmd.com   1/1/12

Improve Your Kidney Health with Dr. Rich Snyder, DO   11/21/11

Glendale Community College Gaucho Gazette   8/22/11

The NephCure Foundation   8/21/11

Authors Show Radio   8/8/11

Renal Support Network: Another 30 Years   1/11/10

Working with Chronic Illness: Are You Aching to Write   1/11/10

I'm going to keep today's blog very short so you have the time to listen to any of the podcasts and/or read any of the articles. When I was teaching college, my students thoroughly enjoyed the time to choose what they'd like to hear or read from a prescribed list. I hope it's the same for you.

4/22/19 *Oh, the Places You'll Go!*

Thank you to Dr. Seuss for lending us the title of today's blog. Oh, you haven't heard of him yet? According to Encyclopaedia Britannica:

"Dr. Seuss, pseudonym of Theodor Seuss Geisel, (born March 2, 1904, Springfield, Massachusetts, U.S.—died September 24, 1991, La Jolla, California), American writer and illustrator of immensely popular children's books, which were noted for their nonsense words, playful rhymes, and unusual creatures."

And why begin the blog with the title of his book you ask. Last month, I received an email from booknowmed.com. Now, I'm not endorsing this new company since I'm not on dialysis and so have not made use of their services myself. However, after reading about the difficulties my dialysis readers were having finding a clinic while they traveled, I was intrigued. Could this be another way to lessen the burden of being on dialysis?

This is from that email:

"What is bookmednow?

Whether you travel for holidays or for work, with booknowmed.com you can now find dialysis clinics that have availability for your treatment dates and book your treatments on the spot, anywhere in the World. And most importanty, booknowmed.com is FREE for patients.

- Browse 440+ dialysis centers, in 380 destinations across 5 continents.

- Find clinics that have availability based on your search criteria.

- Know the price of treatment, before booking.
- See ratings and read reviews from previous patients at the clinic.
- Book your treatments on the spot in safety.
- No booking fees, no hidden costs.
- Track the progress of your booking, directly from your account.

Booknowmed.com is supported by the European Union and 60 national Kidney Patient Associations globally."

Based on this alone, I asked Vassia Efstathiou, the User Experience Manager, if she'd be interested in guest blogging… and she was. This is what she had to say, with just a bit of editing from me.

"Free booking engine for dialysis treatments? Dream or reality?

Travelling while on dialysis is a challenge on its own. Consider having to research, book and coordinate your dialysis treatments abroad. This process can be particularly stressful for dialysis patients, especially when faced with language barriers, lack of information - like the availability of clinics and cost of treatments- and, of course, safety concerns.

Many dialysis patients know this already but the power of the Internet alone cannot do much in this case. So it is definitely good news to hear that the first booking engine for holiday dialysis is live, and even better news to see that it actually works. Let alone the fact that it is free for patients!

Since its launch, thousands of dialysis patients have used booknowmed.com to book more than 27,000 treatments around the globe.

booknowmed.com allows dialysis patients to browse, find and book their dialysis treatments anywhere in the World. We are talking literally - anywhere.

By visiting booknowmed.com you will be able to browse more than 450 dialysis centers in 380 destinations, across five continents. This includes standard holiday options like Spain, Greece, and Turkey, as well some less ordinary destinations like Bali, Sri Lanka, Miami, Brazil and Argentina. Cuba, Barbados, and Curacao are coming up this month.

Bookings are completely free for patients, meaning there are no booking or other hidden costs. Overall the platform is very user-friendly and the booking process is very simple:

1. Patients select their treatment dates and desired destination.

2. They are then presented with a list of the clinics that match their search criteria and - most importantly - have availability for the requested dates.

3. Booking is completed after a simple registration process, which is there for safety reasons. The process takes three minutes and includes registering the patient's full name, email, and telephone number.

But let's examine what differentiates booknowmed.com to the online directories currently available to dialysis patients.

Firstly, we are talking about a booking engine where you can book your treatments on the spot. In contrast to online directories, booknowmed.com allows you to know the availability and price before booking. You can select your exact treatment dates and preferred shift, and complete your booking without picking up the phone or waiting for a reply that takes weeks. Consider that the average booking time on booknowmed.com is six minutes compare to 15 days, the average booking time when you contact the clinic directly or go through a directory service.

Secondly, you have a wide variety of options to choose from, not only in terms of destination but also in terms of the type of the medical facility. booknowmed.com offers the largest network of independent dialysis centers. From global leaders - like Diaverum - to public and private hospitals as well as independent state-of-the-art clinics around the globe.

Thirdly, the simplicity of the booking process itself.

And last, but definitely not least, the great features offered to patients, which promote transparency and allow them to have all the information in hand before booking. These include:

- Know the price of treatment before booking.

- Use smart filters to narrow down your research. If you are an EU patient, for example, you can select to be presented with only the clinics that accept the EHIC.

- See ratings and read reviews written by real patients who have completed treatment at this particular clinic.

- Track the progress of your booking through your account. All the details of the booking including the exact time

- frame of the treatment, contact details of the clinic, and even a map with instructions on how to get there can be found in your account.

booknowmed.com was created by professionals with years of expertise in renal healthcare and the goal to serve a true need for patients. It has received the support of the European Union as well as of national kidney patient associations globally.

The company has plans to expand the functionalities of the platform, with the goal to become a 360o platform serving various everyday needs of renal patients, from nutrition and supplements to an online database and the online exchange of medical reports.

booknowmed.com is the living proof that we have entered a new era for dialysis patients, who can now find and book treatments abroad, with no hassle, no risk, and no language barriers.

Gail here, hoping this is exactly what you've been looking for to make your travel while on dialysis an easier experience for you.

## 4/29/19 *Chemo and My Kidneys*

As most of you know, I am extremely protective of my kidneys. When I was first diagnosed with Chronic Kidney Disease 11 years ago, my eGFR was only 39. Here's a quick reminder of what the eGFR is from my first CKD book, ***What Is It and How Did I Get It? Early Stage Chronic Kidney Disease***:

"GFR: Glomerular filtration rate [if there is a lower case 'e' before the term, it means estimated glomerular filtration rate] which determines both the stage of kidney disease and how well the kidneys are functioning."

39. That's stage 3B, the lower part of stage 3B. During the intervening 11 years, I've been able to raise it to 50 (and sometimes higher for short periods) via vigorously following the renal diet, exercising, avoiding stress as much as possible, maintaining adequate sleep, and paying strict attention to the medications prescribed for me. While the medications were the ones I had been taking for high blood pressure prior to being diagnosed with CKD, they worked in my favor.

This excerpt from The National Center for Biotechnology Information (NCBI) part of the United States National Library of Medicine (NLM), a branch of the National Institutes of Health (NIH) will explain why:

"The decision of whether to reduce blood pressure levels in someone who has chronic kidney disease will depend on

- how high their blood pressure is (when untreated),
- whether they have diabetes, and
- how much protein is in their urine (albumin level).

A person with normal blood pressure who doesn't have diabetes and hardly has any albumin in their urine will be able to get by without using any blood-pressure-lowering medication. But people who have high blood pressure, diabetes or high levels of albumin in their urine are advised to have treatment with ACE inhibitors (angiotensin-converting enzyme inhibitors) or sartans (angiotensin receptor blockers). In people who have diabetes, blood-sugar-lowering medication is also important."

When I was first diagnosed with pancreatic cancer early last month, it changed my medical priorities. With my nephrologist's blessing, my primary focus was the cancer… not my kidneys. It took constant reminders to myself not to be so quick to say no to anything that I thought would harm my kidneys. In other words, to those things I'd been saying no to for the last 11 years.

For example, once diagnosed with CKD, I ate very little protein keeping to my five ounce daily limitation. Not anymore. Protein is needed to avoid muscle wasting during chemotherapy with a minimum requirement of eight ounces a day. I even tried roast beef and other red meats. After 11 years, they no longer agreed with me so I eat ground turkey, chicken, cheese, and am considering soy.

Another change: I preferred not to eat carbohydrates, but was warned not to lose weight if I could help it. All of a sudden I'm eating Goldfish, bread, and pasta. I can't say that I'm enjoying them, but I am keeping my weight loss to a minimum. Other limitations like those on potassium and phosphorous have also gone by the wayside. I've eaten every childhood favorite, foods that I've avoided for the last 11 years, and anything that might look tempting in the last month, but none of them really taste that good. I like the foods on the renal diet now.

Oh, the only thing I have not increased is salt. My daughter takes me to my chemotherapy sessions. There's a Jewish style restaurant across the street and we showed up early one day. I wanted to try a toasted bagel with butter, the way I ate it before CKD. The damned thing was salty! I hadn't expected that.

Back to chemo and my kidneys. I admit it. I was nervous. What was this combination of poisons going to do to my kidneys? If it was so caustic that I had to have a port in place so that it wouldn't be injected directly into my veins for fear of obliterating them, what about my kidneys?

I anxiously awaited my first Comprehensive Blood Panel, the blood test that includes your GFR. Oh, oh, oh! My kidney function had risen to 55 and my creatinine had lowered to 1.0. Let me explain just how good this was.

A GFR of 55 is the higher part of stage 3A. 60 is where stage 2 of CKD begins. My kidneys were functioning better on chemo. And the creatinine? Let's get a quick definition of that first. According to The National Institute of Diabetes and Digestive and Kidney Diseases:

"Creatinine. Creatinine is a waste product from the normal breakdown of muscles in your body. Your kidneys remove creatinine from your blood. Providers use the amount of creatinine in your blood to estimate your GFR. As kidney disease gets worse, the level of creatinine goes up."

Yet, mine went down. How? I asked and it was explained that all the hydration used to clear my veins of the caustic chemotherapy had worked this magic. I had two hours of hydration before the chemotherapy itself, two hours afterward, and another two hours the next day. My kidneys had never been this hydrated!

But wait, there's more. I have diabetes. The pancreas is the organ that produces insulin. Could my diabetes be from the tumor blocking the production of insulin by my pancreas? I truly don't know, but my glucose level is within the standard range for the first time since I've been diagnosed with diabetes.

Would I recommend chemotherapy to raise your GFR, and lower your creatinine and your glucose level? Of course not. But I am feeling so very lucky that my kidneys are not coming to any harm during the chemotherapy necessary to save my life. I can't begin to tell you how relieved I am.

## 5/6/19 *That's Not a Kind of Kidney Disease. Or Is It?*

It's like I'm attuned to anything kidney. After eleven years of writing about Chronic Kidney Disease, I'll bet I am. Sometimes, it's the smallest connection that triggers something in my mind. For example, Sjögren's syndrome kept nagging at me, although I'd never heard of it as a sort of kidney disease. So, what was it and what did it have to do with the kidneys? I went right to the Sjögren's Syndrome Foundation for information.

**"Sjögren's & Kidney Disease**

*by Philip L. Cohen, MD, Professor of Medicine, Temple University School of Medicine*

About 5% of people with Sjögren's develop kidney problems. In most of these patients, the cause is inflammation around the kidney tubules, where urine is collected, concentrated, and becomes acidic. The infiltrating blood cells (mostly lymphocytes) injure the tubular cells, so that the urine does not become as acidic as it should. This condition, called distal renal tubular acidosis, is frequently asymptomatic, but can cause excessive potassium to be excreted in the urine, and may lead to kidney stones or (very rarely) low enough blood potassium to cause muscle weakness or heart problems. Very occasionally, injury to the renal tubules can cause impairment in the ability to concentrate urine, leading to excessive urine volume and increased drinking of fluids (nephrogenic diabetes insipidus).

A smaller number of patients with Sjögren's may develop inflammation of the glomeruli, which are the tiny capillaries through which blood is filtered to produce urine. This may cause protein to leak into the urine, along with red blood cells. Sometimes a kidney biopsy is needed to establish the exact diagnosis and treatment. Treatment options may include corticosteroids and immunosuppressive drugs to prevent loss of kidney function.

This information was first printed in *The Moisture Seekers*, SSF's patient newsletter for members."

This reminds me of when I was teaching critical thinking on the college level. First, we'd hit the class with an article about something foreign to them and then, we'd show them how to figure out what it meant. For our purposes, a few explanations might be a good place to start.

Tubules, huh? What are those? Actually, the word just means tube shaped. Remembering that renal and kidney mean the same thing, we can see the problem area.

Now remember, CKD patients are usually limited as to how much fluid they can drink per day. Too much forces the kidneys to work too hard to clear the urine from your body. Remember the car analogy from **What Is It and How Did I Get It? Early Stage Chronic Kidney Disease**?

As for potassium, that's one of the electrolytes CKD patients need to be aware of. This article by Dr. Parker on Healthy Way explains:

"Potassium does many important functions in the body. This essential mineral is mainly found inside the cells of our body. Low potassium levels are associated with many health conditions including hypertension, irregular heartbeat, and muscle weakness. We should take adequate amounts of potassium-rich foods for a healthy life.

**Potassium is essential for the heart**

We need potassium to maintain the blood pressure within normal range. There should be a balance between sodium and potassium in the body to regulate our blood pressure. Too much sodium and too little potassium can elevate your blood pressure.

In addition, potassium is needed for the contraction of the heart. Potassium levels in the blood should be kept nearly constant or within a narrow range for the proper pumping action of the heart. The heart may stop beating if we have high or low levels of potassium in the blood.

**We need potassium for stronger muscles**

Most of the potassium in the body is found inside the muscle cells. It is the main positively charged ion inside the cells. It is essential for the contraction of muscles. Low levels of potassium are associated with muscle twitching, cramps and muscle weakness. Very low levels can cause paralysis of the muscles.

Hypokalemic periodic paralysis is a disorder that causes occasional episodes of muscle weakness and paralysis caused by lower levels of potassium in the blood. It is a genetic condition that runs in families.

**It is essential for nerve conduction**

Sodium and potassium are needed to maintain the electrical potential across the nerve cells. This electrical charge is essential for the conduction of nerve signals along the nerves. It protects from stroke.

Researchers found eating potassium-rich foods is associated with reduced incidents of stroke. A recent study conducted in postmenopausal women supports the findings. One of the co-researchers says, 'post-menopausal women should eat more potassium-rich foods, such as fruits, vegetables, beans, milk and unprocessed meats in order to lower their risk of stroke and death'.

**It is important for water and electrolyte balance in the body**

Water and electrolyte balance is maintained by the kidneys. This is one of the important functions of the kidneys. Aldosterone, a hormone secreted by the adrenal glands plays the primary role in the balance of sodium and potassium.

The normal blood level of potassium is 3.5 to 5 mmol/l. A level of less than 3.5 is called hypokalemia, and more than 5 is called hyperkalemia. To achieve the normal blood level, we need to take about 4 to 5 grams of potassium per day. An average size banana will provide about 25% of daily requirement.

It is recommended to eat foods that have plenty of potassium. In addition, your diet should contain low amounts of sodium (salt). Taking supplements is not a good idea. It can cause many side effects.

People who have certain medical conditions such as chronic kidney failure should not eat large amounts of potassium-rich foods.

People who take certain types of medications should consult a doctor about their potassium intake. Some may need additional intake while others may need to restrict the intake of potassium rich foods."

So, while Sjögren's syndrome may not be a kind of kidney disease, it can affect your kidneys. Thanks for keeping me company while I made the connection for myself.

## 5/13/19 *Don't Know Much about FSGS...*

Being on chemotherapy is very tiring, so I stay home a lot and delve into anything that catches my eye, like FSGS. I've seen the letters before and had sort of a vague idea of what it might be, but what better time to explore it and whatever it may have to do with Chronic Kidney Disease than now?

Let's start at the beginning. FSGS is the acronym for focal segmental glomerulosclerosis. Anything look familiar? Maybe the 'glomerul' part of glomerulosclerosis? I think we need to know the definition of glomerulosclerosis to be able to answer that question. The National Institutes of Health's U.S. National Library of Congress's Medline Plus defines it this way:

"Focal segmental glomerulosclerosis is scar tissue in the filtering unit of the kidney. This structure is called the glomerulus. The glomeruli serve as filters that help the body get rid of harmful substances. Each kidney has thousands of glomeruli.

'Focal' means that some of the glomeruli become scarred. Others remain normal. 'Segmental' means that only part of an individual glomerulus is damaged."

So, we do know what the 'glomerul' part of glomerulosclerosis means. It refers to the same filters in the kidneys we've been discussing for the past eleven years: the glomeruli. This former English teacher can assure you that 'o' is simply a connective between the two parts of the word. 'Sclerosis' is a term you may have heard of in relation to the disease of the same name, the one in which the following occurs (according to Encarta Dictionary):

"the hardening and thickening of body tissue as a result of unwarranted growth, degeneration of nerve fibers, or deposition of minerals, especially calcium."

Wait a minute. When I first started writing about CKD, I approached NephCure Foundation... not being certain what it was, but seeing Neph in its name. They were kind enough to ask me to guest blog for them on 8/21/11. By the way, as of August 15, 2014, NephCure Foundation became NephCure Kidney International. That makes the connection to our kidneys much more clear.

Back to FSGS. NephCure Kidney International offers us this information:

"How is FSGS Diagnosed?

FSGS is diagnosed with renal biopsy (when doctors examine a tiny portion of the kidney tissue), however, because only some sections of the glomeruli are affected, the biopsy can sometimes be inconclusive.

What are the Symptoms of FSGS?

Many people with FSGS have no symptoms at all. When symptoms are present the most common include:

**Proteinuria** – Large amounts of protein 'spilling' into the urine

**Edema** – Swelling in parts of the body, most noticeable around the eyes, hands and feet, and abdomen which causes sudden weight gain.

**Low Blood Albumin Levels** because the kidneys are removing albumin instead of returning it to the blood

**High Cholesterol** in some cases

**High Blood Pressure** in some cases and can often be hard to treat

FSGS can also cause abnormal results of creatinine in laboratory tests. Creatinine is measured by taking a blood sample. Everyone has a certain amount of a substance called creatinine floating in his or her blood. This substance is always being produced by healthy muscles and normally the kidneys constantly filter it out and the level of creatinine stays low. But when the filters become damaged, they stop filtering properly and the level of creatinine left in the blood goes up."

Whoa! Look at all the terms we've used again and again in the last eleven years of ***SlowItDownCKD***'s weekly blog: proteinuria, edema, albumin, cholesterol, high blood pressure, and creatinine. This is definitely something that we, as CKD patients, should know about.

Okay. Let's say you are diagnosed with FSGS. Now what? The National Kidney Organization was helpful here:

**"How is FSGS treated?**

The type of treatment you get depends on the cause. Everyone is different and your doctor will make a treatment plan that is right for your type of FSGS. Usually, treatments for FSGS include:

- Corticosteroids (often called "steroids")
- Immunosuppressive drugs
- ACE inhibitors and ARBs

- Diuretics

- Diet change

Corticosteroids and immunosuppressive drugs: These medications are used to calm your immune system (your body's defense system) and stop it from attacking your glomeruli.

ACE inhibitors and ARBs: These are blood pressure medications used to reduce protein loss and control blood pressure.

Diuretics: These medications help your body get rid of excess fluid and swelling. These can be used to lower your blood pressure too.

Diet changes: Some diet changes may be needed, such as reducing salt (sodium) and protein in your food choices to lighten the load of wastes on the kidneys."

I think we need another definition here. It's Plasmapheresis. Back to the Encarta Dictionary.

"a process in which blood taken from a patient is treated to extract the cells and corpuscles, which are then added to another fluid and returned to the patient's body."

Let's go back to NephCure Kidney International for a succinct summary of FSGS Facts.

"More than 5400 patients are diagnosed with FSGS every year, however, this is considered an underestimate because:

- a limited number of biopsies are performed

- the number of FSGS cases are rising more than any other cause of Nephrotic Syndrome…

NephCure estimates that there are currently 19,306 people living with ESRD due to FSGS..., in part because it is the most common cause of steroid resistant Nephrotic Syndrome in children... and it is the second leading cause of kidney failure in children...

NephCure estimates that people of African ancestry are at a five times higher diagnosis rate of FSGS...

About half of FSGS patients who do not respond to steroids go into ESRD each year, requiring dialysis or transplantation...

Approximately 1,000 FSGS patients a year receive kidney transplants... however, within hours to weeks after a kidney transplant, FSGS returns in approximately 30-40% of patients...."

As prevalent and serious as this sounds, please remember that FSGS is a rare kidney disease. Knowing what we now know just may help you keep your eyes open for it.

## 5/20/19 *Clinical Trials Day*

By now, you probably all know that I chose a clinical trial to treat my pancreatic cancer. But did you know that today, May 20th, is Clinical Trials Day? (Just so you know, I've included this particular blog in **SlowItDownCKD 2019** even though the event has passed because it's Clinical Trials Day every year.)

What's that, you ask? Let's find out together. According to The Association of Clinical Research Professionals (ACRP):

"WHY MAY 20?

Clinical Trials Day is celebrated around the world in May to recognize the day that James Lind started what is often considered the first randomized clinical trial aboard a ship on May 20, 1747.

HERE'S THE STORY

May, 1747.

The HMS Salisbury of Britain's Royal Navy fleet patrols the English Channel at a time when scurvy is thought to have killed more British seamen than French and Spanish arms.

Aboard this ship, surgeon mate James Lind, a pioneer of naval hygiene, conducts what many refer to as the first clinical trial.

Acting on a hunch that scurvy was caused by putrefaction of the body that could be cured through the introduction of acids, Lind recruited 12 men for his 'fair test.'...

From The James Lind Library:

*Without stating what method of allocation he used, Lind allocated two men to each of six different daily treatments for a period of fourteen days. The six treatments were: 1.1 litres of cider; twenty-five millilitres of elixir vitriol (dilute sulphuric acid); 18 millilitres of vinegar three times throughout the day before meals; half a pint of sea water; two oranges and one lemon continued for six days only (when the supply was exhausted); and a medicinal paste made up of garlic, mustard seed, dried radish root and gum myrrh....*

Those allocated citrus fruits experienced 'the most sudden and good visible effects,' according to Lind's report on the trial.

Though Lind, according to The James Lind Library, might have left his readers 'confused about his recommendations' regarding the use of citrus in curing scurvy, he is 'rightly recognized for having taken care to 'compare like with like,' and the design of his trial may have inspired 'and informed future clinical trial design.'"

I've written about James Lind before, so you may want to re-read the 8/20/18 blog to read more about him and his experiments.

\*\*\*

"Headline: Chronic Kidney Disease Research: How to Get Involved

By Nancy Ryerson

May 20 is Clinical Trials Day. Every year, patient advocates and research groups participate to raise awareness of how clinical trial participation drives research progress. You may know that new treatments for Chronic Kidney Disease (CKD) can't move forward without clinical trial volunteers, but you may not know how to find active, relevant trials in your area.

Below, you'll find answers to commonly asked questions about finding CKD clinical trials, including who can join, how to find trials, and the kinds of questions CKD research aims to answer.

**How can I find Chronic Kidney Disease clinical trials near me?**

…. All clinical trials are listed on ClinicalTrials.gov, but because the website was developed with researchers in mind rather than patients, it can be difficult for patients to navigate. Antidote is a clinical trial matching company that provides a patient-friendly clinical trial search tool to health nonprofits and bloggers, including this blog. With the Antidote tool, you can answer a few questions about your medical history and where you'd like to find a trial to receive a list of trials you may qualify for in your area. You can also sign up to receive alerts when new trials are added near you.

**Who can join CKD clinical trials?**

It's a common misconception that clinical trials only need volunteers who have been recently diagnosed to take part. It's also untrue that clinical trials are only a 'last resort' for patients who have exhausted other options. In reality, clinical trials can be a care option for patients at any point after diagnosis. CKD trials need volunteers with mild, moderate, and severe kidney disease to participate in different trials. Some trials also look for patients with specific comorbidities, such as hypertension.

**What does CKD research typically focus on?**

Clinical trials for Chronic Kidney Disease (CKD) research potential new treatments to slow or stop CKD, as well as treat common conditions associated with CKD, such as anemia or hypertension. CKD clinical trials aren't limited to research into new drugs, either. For example, a kidney-friendly diet can make a significant difference in reducing kidney damage, and more research is needed into specific interventions that can help. Research studies are also looking into the impact exercise can have on CKD symptoms and progression.

Clinical trials may also be observational. These kinds of trials don't test an intervention – a drug, diet, lifestyle change, etc. Instead, participants are divided into groups and observed for differences in outcome.

**Do clinical trials always use a placebo?**

In clinical trials, placebos – also known as 'sugar pills' – help researchers understand the effectiveness of an experimental treatment. While they can be an important part of the research process, it's also understandable that patients hope they won't receive the placebo in a clinical trial.

If you're considering taking part in a trial but you're concerned about receiving a placebo, it's important to know that not all trials use one. Many trials test a potential new treatment against the standard of care, for example. In some trials that use a placebo, everyone in the trial may receive the study drug at some point during the trial.

**I don't have time to participate in a clinical trial.**

Time restraints are another reason many patients hesitate to participate in clinical trials. While some clinical trials may require weekly site visits, others may only ask participants to come in every month or so. Some trials may also offer virtual visits online or home visits to help reduce the number of trips you'll need to take to get to a site. When you're considering joining a clinical trial, ask the study team any questions you have about the trial schedule, reimbursement for travel, or anything else about participation."

Interested in finding a trial near you? Use the ***SlowItDownCKD*** trial search, powered by Antidote, to start your search. It's near the middle on the right side of the blog. Ladies and Gentleman, start your motors! I hope you find just the right CKD Clinical Trial for you.

## 5/27/19 *No Longer a Transfusion Virgin*

I've been thinking about the similarities between Chronic Kidney Disease treatment and Pancreatic Cancer treatment... or, at least, my Pancreatic Cancer treatment. Some are superficial, like going to the Research Institute several days a week for chemotherapy and those on dialysis going to the dialysis center several days a week for dialysis.

Some are not. A current topic of similarity was an eye opener for me. I am 72 years old and have never had a transfusion before last Monday. I'd gone to the Research Institute where I'm part of a clinical trial for a simple non-chemotherapy day checkup. This supposedly two hour appointment turned into almost eight hours. Why?

If you can understand these labs, you'll know. If not, no problem. You know I'll explain.

| Component | Your Value | Standard Range |
|---|---|---|
| **RBC** | **2.23** $10^{\wedge}6/uL$ | *3.50 – 5.40 $10^{\wedge}6/uL$* |
| **Hemoglobin** | **6.8** g/dL | *12.0 – 16.0 g/dL* |
| **Hematocrit** | **19.7** % | *36.0 – 48.0 %* |
| **RDW** | **16.0** % | *11.5 – 14.5 %* |
| **Platelets** | **15** K/uL | *130 – 450 K/uL* |

Let's start at the top of the list. RBC stands for red blood cells.

MedicineNet tells us:

"Red blood cells: The blood cells that carry oxygen. Red cells contain hemoglobin and it is the hemoglobin which permits them to transport oxygen (and carbon dioxide). Hemoglobin, aside from being a transport molecule, is a pigment. It gives the cells their red color (and their name).

The abbreviation for red blood cells is RBCs. Red blood cells are sometime simply called red cells. They are also called erythrocytes or, rarely today, red blood corpuscles."

So it makes sense that if RBC is below the standard range (column on the right), the hemoglobin will also be. And where are RBCs produced? Let's trot on over to the National Institute of Diabetes, Digestive, and Kidney Disease (NIKKD) for the answer to that one:

"Healthy kidneys produce a hormone called erythropoietin (EPO). A hormone is a chemical produced by the body and released into the blood to help trigger or regulate particular body functions. EPO prompts the bone marrow to make red blood cells, which then carry oxygen throughout the body.

**What causes anemia in chronic kidney disease?**

When kidneys are diseased or damaged, they do not make enough EPO. As a result, the bone marrow makes fewer red blood cells, causing anemia. When blood has fewer red blood cells, it deprives the body of the oxygen it needs."

Now, this is not saying all CKD patients will have anemia, although it is common is the later stages of the disease. Chemotherapy had a lot to do with this, too.

What about this hematocrit? What is that? I went to the University of Rochester's Health Encyclopedia for help here:

"This test measures how much of your blood is made up of red blood cells.

Normal blood contains white blood cells, red blood cells, platelets, and the fluid portion called plasma. The word *hematocrit* means *to separate*. In this test, your red blood cells are separated from the rest of your blood so they can be measured.

Your hematocrit (HCT) shows whether you have a normal amount of red blood cells, too many, or too few. To measure your HCT, your blood sample is spun at a high speed to separate the red blood cells."

MedicalNewsToday helps us understand the RDW or red cell distribution width:

"If the results of a CBC [Gail here: that's the complete blood count.] show low levels of red blood cells or hemoglobin, this usually suggests anemia. Doctors will then try to determine the cause of the condition using the RDW and other tests."

So, we're back to anemia. By the way, cancer is one of the diseases that can cause high numbers on your RDW. CKD is not, but diabetes – one of the primary causes of CKD – is.

I added platelets to the list since they are such an integral part of your blood. MedLinePlus explains succinctly (time for me to find other words for succinctly) just what they are and what they do:

"Platelets, also known as thrombocytes, are small pieces of blood cells. They form in your bone marrow, a sponge-like tissue in your bones. Platelets play a major role in blood clotting. Normally, when one of your blood vessels is injured, you start to bleed. Your platelets will clot (clump together) to plug the hole in the blood vessel and stop the bleeding. You can have different problems with your platelets:

If your blood has a low number of platelets, it is called thrombocytopenia. This can put you at risk for mild to serious bleeding. The bleeding could be external or internal. There can be various causes. If the problem is mild, you may not need treatment. For more serious cases, you may need medicines or blood or platelet transfusions…."

I had my second infusion of platelets along with my first transfusion last week.

I've offered a multitude of definitions today. The point here is that both CKD patients and chemotherapy patients (and others suffering from a host of maladies) may need transfusions.

Right. I haven't discussed what a transfusion is yet. Dictionary.com defines it a little simplistically for us:

"the direct transferring of blood, plasma, or the like into a blood vessel."

The MayoClinic adds:

"Your blood will be tested before a transfusion to determine whether your blood type is A, B, AB or O and whether your blood is Rh positive or Rh negative. The donated blood used for your transfusion must be compatible with your blood type."

6/3/19 *More Time to Learn*

I don't think I've ever felt this tired in my life. Cancer does that... and it leaves me a lot of time in bed to explore whatever I'd like to on the internet. So now I'm discovering all these – what's the word? – possibly peripheral? diseases that affect the kidneys. For example, while I don't have the energy to post a new Chronic Kidney Disease picture on Instagram every day, I do check the site daily and like what appeals to me and learn from what's new to me.

That's where I noticed posts about Bartter syndrome. If you're like me, you want to know about something you've never heard of before. Let's explore this together.

I went directly to my old friend, MedlinePlus, which is part of the U.S. National Library of Medicine for a definition and the causes:

"Bartter syndrome is a group of rare conditions that affect the kidneys.

**Causes**

There are five gene defects known to be associated with Bartter syndrome. The condition is present at birth (congenital). The condition is caused by a defect in the kidneys' ability to reabsorb sodium. People affected by Bartter syndrome lose too much sodium through the urine. This causes a rise in the level of the hormone aldosterone, and makes the kidneys remove too much potassium from the body. This is known as potassium wasting. The condition also results in an abnormal acid balance in the blood called hypokalemic alkalosis, which causes too much calcium in the urine."

It looks like there are a few terms here we may not be familiar with. Let's take a look at aldosterone. The Hormone Health Network from the Endocrine Society tells us:

"Aldosterone is produced in the cortex of the adrenal glands, which are located above the kidneys.... Aldosterone affects the body's ability to regulate blood pressure. It sends the signal to organs, like the kidney and colon, that can increase the amount of sodium the body sends into the bloodstream or the amount of potassium released in the urine. The hormone also causes the bloodstream to re-absorb water with the sodium to increase blood volume. All of these actions are integral to increasing and lowering blood vessels. Indirectly, the hormone also helps maintain the blood's pH and electrolyte levels."

And hypokalemic alkalosis? What is that? Healthline gave me the answer:

"**Hypokalemic alkalosis**

Hypokalemic alkalosis occurs when your body lacks the normal amount of the mineral potassium. You normally get potassium from your food, but not eating enough of it is rarely the cause of a potassium deficiency. Kidney disease, excessive sweating, and diarrhea are just a few ways you can lose too much potassium. Potassium is essential to the proper functioning of the:

- heart
- kidneys
- muscles
- nervous system

- digestive system"

Hmmm, so kidney disease can cause you to lose too much potassium, which can then interfere with the proper functioning of your kidneys. Doesn't sound good to me. But, remember that the condition is congenital and will show up at birth.

Let's say it does. Then what? According to Verywellhealth:

"Treatment of Bartter syndrome focuses on keeping the blood potassium at a normal level. This is done by having a diet rich in potassium and taking potassium supplements if needed. There are also drugs that reduce the loss of potassium in the urine, such as spironolactone, triamterene, or amiloride. Other medications used to treat Bartter syndrome may include indomethacin, captopril, and in children, growth hormone."

Food rich in potassium? I'm sure bananas came directly into your mind but there are others. I chose to use the National Kidney Foundation's list of high potassium foods since this is a blog about CKD.

**"What foods are high in potassium (greater than 200 milligrams per portion)?**

The following table lists foods that are high in potassium. The portion size is ½ cup unless otherwise stated. Please be sure to check portion sizes. While all the foods on this list are high in potassium, some are higher than others.

## High-Potassium Foods

| Fruits | Vegetables | Other Foods |
|---|---|---|
| Apricot, raw (2 medium) dried (5 halves) | Acorn Squash | Bran/Bran products |
| Avocado (¼ whole) | Artichoke | Chocolate (1.5-2 ounces) |
| Banana (½ whole) | Bamboo Shoots | Granola |
| Cantaloupe | Baked Beans | Milk, all types (1 cup) |
| Dates (5 whole) | Butternut Squash | Molasses (1 Tablespoon) |
| Dried fruits | Refried Beans | Nutritional Supplements: Use only under the direction of your doctor or dietitian. |
| Figs, dried | Beets, fresh then boiled | |
| Grapefruit Juice | Black Beans | |
| Honeydew | Broccoli, cooked | Nuts and Seeds (1 ounce) |
| Kiwi (1 medium) | Brussels Sprouts | Peanut Butter (2 tbs.) |
| Mango (1 medium) | Chinese Cabbage | Salt Substitutes/Lite Salt |

| | | |
|---|---|---|
| Orange (1 medium) | Dried Beans and Peas | Yogurt |
| Orange Juice | Greens, except Kale | Snuff/Chewing Tobacco |
| Papaya (½ whole) | Hubbard Squash | |
| Pomegranate (1 whole) | Kohlrabi | |
| Pomegranate Juice | Lentils | |
| Prunes | Legumes | |
| Prune Juice | White Mushrooms, cooked (½ cup) | |
| Raisins | Okra | |
| | Parsnips | |
| | Potatoes, white and sweet | |
| | Pumpkin | |
| | Rutabagas | |
| | Spinach, cooked | |
| | Tomatoes/Tomato products | |

Vegetable Juices"

I also have a list of food sensitivities, so I avoid those foods. If you do, too, you might want to cross those foods off your high potassium foods list if you just happen to have Bartter syndrome.

## 6/10/19 *Like Life?*

A word I hear every few weeks at chemotherapy is Neulasta. I looked it up since I was being given an injection each time I heard the word. I went directly to the manufacturer's website to find out just what it was:

"Neulasta® is a prescription medicine used to help reduce the chance of infection due to a low white blood cell count, in people with certain types of cancer (non-myeloid), who receive anti-cancer medicines (chemotherapy) that can cause fever and low blood cell count."

But then I needed to define 'non-myeloid' for myself. No problem. I called up my old standby The Merriam-Webster Dictionary:

"not being, involving, or affecting bone marrow"

Okay, got it. Neulasta reduces low white blood cell count infection in cancer that doesn't affect the bone marrow. By the way, this is accomplished by forcing white blood cells – the infection fighting blood cells – to mature quickly.

No sooner did I get that straight in my mind than I started hearing a different word: Udenyca. It turned out that Udenya is a biosimilar for Neulasta. Now we get to the meat of the matter.

Just what is a biosimilar? I took a former English teacher's stab at the definition and decided it meant 'like life.' But does it? The Free Medical Dictionary helped us out here:

"biosimilar (bī′ō-sĭm′ə-lər) *adj.*

Highly similar in function and effect to an existing biological product, especially to a biologic that has already been clincaly tested and approved for use.

*n.*

A biological product that is biosimilar to an existing product, especially to a biologic"

Keep in mind that an adjective (adj.) describes a noun, while a noun (n.) is a person, place, thing, or idea.

Frankly, I didn't find this very helpful. So I did what I considered the logical thing and looked to the Food and Drug Administration (FDA) for more explanation:

"A biosimilar is a biological product

FDA-approved biosimilars have been compared to an FDA-approved biologic, known as the reference product. Reference and biosimilar products are:

Large and generally complex molecules

Produced from living organisms

Carefully monitored to ensure consistent quality

Meet FDA's rigorous standards for approval

Are manufactured in FDA-licensed facilities

Are tracked as part of post-market surveillance to ensure continued safety

A biosimilar is highly similar to a reference product

For approval, the structure and function of an approved biosimilar were compared to a reference product, looking at key characteristics such as:

Purity

Molecular structure

Bioactivity

The data from these comparisons must show that the biosimilar is highly similar to the reference product.

A biosimilar has no clinically meaningful differences from a reference product

Studies were performed to show that biosimilars have no clinically meaningful differences in safety, purity or potency (safety and effectiveness) compared to the reference product:

Pharmacokinetic and, if needed, armacodynamic studies

Immunogenicity assessment

Additional clinical studies as needed

Studies may be done independently or combined.

A biosimilar is approved by FDA after rigorous evaluation and testing by the applicant

Prescribers and patients should have no concerns about using these medications instead of reference products because biosimilars:

Meet FDA's rigorous standards for approval

Are manufactured in FDA-licensed facilities

Are tracked as part of post-market surveillance to ensure continued safety"

Okay! Now we're talking. Pretty simple to understand, isn't it? Well, maybe there's a word or three we might need defined. Let's take another look. These two definitions are from Dictionary.com.

"Pharmacokinetic –
the branch of pharmacology that studies the fate of pharmacologi cal substances in the
body, as their absorption, distribution, metabolism, and elimination.

Immunogenicity –

causing or capable of producing an immune response."

Wikipedia offered this interesting difference between Pharmacokinetic and Pharmacodynamics.

"Pharmacodynamics is the study of how a drug affects an organism, whereas pharmacokinetics is the study of how the organism affects the drug. Both together influence dosing, benefit, and adverse effects."

The point here is that the synthetic drug and biosimilars are not the same. Maybe my guess at their definition is far off the mark. And lest you're beginning to think this is a cancer blog rather than a Chronic Kidney Disease blog, biosimilars are used in CKD, too.

This snippet from the Clinical Journal of the American Society of Nephrology (CJASN) will give you the idea:

"Most recognizable to nephrologists is the biologic recombinant human erythropoietin (rHuEPO). Considerably more expensive to develop and produce, biologics are more structurally complex than small-molecule drugs. By 2020, biologics will constitute an estimated 27% of spending on worldwide pharmacologics."

Remember erythropoietin, more commonly known among CKD patients as epo? Not to worry; MedicineNet will remind us:

"**Erythropoietin** (EPO) is a hormone produced by the kidney that promotes the formation of red blood cells by the bone marrow. The kidney cells that make erythropoietin are sensitive to low oxygen levels in the blood that travels through the kidney."

Un-oh, I almost forgot to explain the difference between biosimilars and biologics. According to the Congressional Research Service:

"A biological product, or biologic, is a preparation, such as a drug or a vaccine, that is made from living organisms. Compared with conventional chemical drugs, biologics are relatively large and complex molecules. They may be composed of proteins (and/or their constituent amino acids), carbohydrates (such as sugars), nucleic acids (such as DNA), or combinations of these substances.

Biologics may also be cells or tissues used in transplantation. A biosimilar, sometimes referred to as a follow-on biologic, is a therapeutic drug that is highly similar but not structurally identical, to a brand-name biologic (i.e., the reference product). This is in contrast to a generic chemical drug, which is an exact copy of a brand-name chemical drug (i.e., the reference listed drug). Because biologics are more complex than chemical drugs, both in composition and method of manufacture, biosimilars will not be exact replicas of the brand-name product, but may instead be shown to be highly similar. However, for many years, the drug industry and the Food and Drug Administration (FDA) have coped with the inherent variability in biological products from natural sources. FDA maintains that the batch-to-batch and lot-to-lot variability that occurs for both brand-name biologics and biosimilars can be assessed and managed effectively."

Hmmm, looks like I've made a fairly simple concept terribly complex.

## 6/17/19 **Platelets Keep It Together**

During my chemo journey, I've needed an infusion of platelets several times. Chronic Kidney Disease patients sometimes need them, too, but I'll write about that later on in this blog. First question from the audience?

Oh, that's a good one: What are platelets? This is from my very first CKD book, ***What Is It and How Did I Get It? Early Stage Chronic Kidney Disease*** and will help to explain.

"1. The white blood cells make up your immune system. There are usually from 7,000 to 25,000 WBC in a drop of blood, but if you have an infection, that number rises since these are the infection fighting blood cells.

2. The red blood cells, also called erythrocytes, carry oxygen to the other cells in your body – so the higher the number here the better – and waste such as carbon dioxide from them. There are approximately five billion red blood cells – the midsized cells – in a single drop of your blood.

3. The platelets deal with the blood's clotting ability by repairing leaks in your blood vessels. Normally, there are 150,000 to 350,000 platelets in one drop of blood."

I've included all three types of blood cells as we just might need that information later on.

Okay, how about another question? What's that? You want to know how you know if your platelets are decreased? When you have blood tests, one of them is usually the CBC or Complete Blood Count. Let's see if we can find more information from The Mayo Clinic.

"A complete blood count (CBC) is a blood test used to evaluate your overall health and detect a wide range of disorders, including anemia, infection and leukemia.

A complete blood count test measures several components and features of your blood, including:

Red blood cells, which carry oxygen

White blood cells, which fight infection

Hemoglobin, the oxygen-carrying protein in red blood cells

Hematocrit, the proportion of red blood cells to the fluid component, or plasma, in your blood

Platelets, which help with blood clotting"

If your doctors are anything like mine, I have one every three months for my primary care doctor, an annual CBC for my nephrologist, and weekly for my oncologist.

Now, remember the normal range of platelets is 150,000 to 350,000 platelets in one drop of blood. Mine were 16,000. Sure, it was the chemotherapy that was killing my platelets, but it was also the chemotherapy that was shrinking the tumor and lowering the tumor markers in my CA19-9 (blood test for tumor markers in pancreatic cancer). I couldn't stop the chemotherapy, but my doctors could raise my platelets via infusion.

Young man in the back? Nice! He wants to know what the difference between infusion and transfusion is. According to The Free Dictionary's Medical Dictionary, infusion means

1. the steeping of a substance in water to obtain its soluble principles.

2. the product obtained by this process.

3. the slow therapeutic introduction of fluid other than blood into a vein.

That's right. The third definition is the one we need.

Using the same source, we learn that transfusion means

"Transfusion is the process of transferring whole blood or blood components from one person (donor) to another (recipient)."

Let's talk about platelet infusions and CKD patients now. UpToDate offers the following, but we may need a bit of hand holding to understand it:

"The association between renal dysfunction and bleeding was recognized more than 200 years ago…. However, there remains an incomplete understanding of the underlying pathophysiology. Impaired platelet function is one of the main determinants of uremic bleeding. This impairment is due largely to incompletely defined inhibitors of platelet function in the plasma of patients with markedly reduced kidney function. Abnormal platelet-endothelial interaction and anemia also play a role."

Do you remember what uremic means? No problem … come along with me to visit my old buddy, the Merriam-Webster Dictionary.

"1: accumulation in the blood of constituents normally eliminated in the urine that produces a severe toxic condition and usually occurs in severe kidney disease

**2:** the toxic bodily condition associated with uremia"

Let's use the same dictionary for the definition of endothelial, which is the adjective or describing word for endothelium.

"1: an epithelium of mesodermal origin composed of a single layer of thin flattened cells that lines internal body cavities and the lumens of vessels

2: the inner layer of the seed coat of some plants"

You guessed it: the first definition is the one we need. I think all the pieces are in place for you to understand the need for the right number of platelets and that platelet infusions are sometimes necessary. Too bad I didn't before my white blouses and nightgowns were stained by the blood leaking from my nose (and other places too delicate to mention). Oh well, I can always buy more clothes.

New topic. I've written about All of Us Research several times and received this email from them this week.

"In case you missed it, we introduced our new Data Browser at the All of Us Research Program symposium on May 6th. The Data Browser is an interactive tool that lets you learn more about the health data that you and all the other participants have contributed so far. Currently in beta testing, it lets you search by topics like health conditions, survey questions, and physical measurements, and will include more data over time.

We invite you to take a look at the Data Browser and let us know what you think. If you have feedback, you can email support@ResearchAllofUs.org."

## 6/24/19 *Diabetic Neuropathy or Not: I WILL Dance Again*

I come from a family of dancers. My parents and their siblings were all light on their feet and danced from the time they were teens right up until just before their deaths. It was a delight to watch them. The tradition continued with me… and my youngest who actually taught blues dancing for several years.

Ah, but then my neuropathy appeared. This was years before the diabetes diagnosis. Hmmm, there's still a question as to whether or not the diabetes was caused by the pancreatic cancer. After all, the pancreas does produce insulin.

I just reread the above two paragraphs and see so much that needs some basic explanation. Let's start with those explanations this week. How many of you know what neuropathy is? I didn't either until I was diagnosed with it. According to my favorite dictionary since college a million years ago, The Merriam-Webster Dictionary defines neuropathy as:

"damage, disease, or dysfunction of one or more nerves especially of the peripheral nervous system that is typically marked by burning or shooting pain, numbness, tingling, or muscle weakness or atrophy, is often degenerative, and is usually caused by injury, infection, disease, drugs, toxins, or vitamin deficiency "

'Peripheral nervous system' means,

"the part of the nervous system that is outside the central nervous system and comprises the cranial nerves excepting the optic nerve, the spinal nerves, and the autonomic nervous system"

Since the neuropathy was so minor before the pancreatic cancer, I wasn't even aware of it until my neurologist did some testing. I knew my feet were tingly sometimes, but I thought they had fallen asleep. It did sort of feel like that.

Then, I started chemotherapy in March. The tingling became so bad that I couldn't feel my feet under me and had to rely on a cane to keep my balance. We thought it was the chemo drugs causing the neuropathy. Uh-oh, that was just about when my hands became affected, too, and my A1C (Remember that one? It's the blood test for the average of your blood glucose over a three month period.) rose all the way to 7.1.

Healthline tells us,

"Someone without diabetes will have about 5 percent of their hemoglobin glycated [Gail here: that means glucose bonded to hemoglobin]. A normal A1C level is 5.6 percent or below, according to the National Institute of Diabetes and Digestive and Kidney Diseases.

A level of 5.7 to 6.4 percent indicates prediabetes. People with diabetes have an A1C level of 6.5 percent or above."

Mind you, during chemotherapy I'd been ordered to eat whatever I could. Getting in the calories would cut down on the expected weight loss. In all honesty, I'm the only person I know what *gained* weight while on chemotherapy.

Now, what is this about the pancreas producing insulin? Might as well get a definition of insulin while we're at it. MedicineNet offered the simplest explanation:

"A natural hormone made by the pancreas that controls the level of the sugar glucose in the blood. Insulin permits cells to use glucose for energy. Cells cannot utilize glucose without insulin."

That would explain why my energy is practically nil, but it also seems to indicate that I won't be able to do anything about it until after the surgery to remove the tumor. Although, when I start radiation next week, I may be able to go back to the diabetic diet. By the way, after following the Chronic Kidney Disease diet for 11 years, none of the new – off the CKD diet – foods I tried are appealing to me.

But I digress. So, what now? I need to dance; it's part of who I am. My oncologist referred me to Occupational Therapy. Now I have exercises and tactile surfaces to explore that may be helpful. But what about those who are not going through chemotherapy, but do have diabetic neuropathy? Remember diabetes is the number one cause of CKD.

Oh, my goodness. It looks like there are as many ways to treat neuropathy as there are different kinds of neuropathy. I hadn't expected that. EverydayHealth gives us an idea of just how complicated choosing the proper treatment for your neuropathy can be:

**"What Are the Main Ways That Neuropathy Is Treated?**

Treating neuropathy in general focuses first on identifying and then addressing the underlying condition to help prevent further damage and give nerves the time they need to heal to the extent that they can.

'The treatment for the neuropathy is to reverse whatever it is that is causing the neuropathy,' says Clifford Segil, DO, a neurologist at Providence Saint John's Health Center in Santa Monica, California. 'We try to reverse the insult to the nerves first and then do symptomatic control.'

For people with diabetic neuropathy, the first step physicians take is getting the person's blood glucose level under control, says Matthew Villani, DPM, a podiatrist at Central Florida Regional Hospital in Sanford, Florida.

This treatment approach aims to remove the 'insult' created by the excess sugar to peripheral nerves throughout the body — but especially the extremities, Dr. Segil explains.

Here are some other ways diabetic neuropathy may be treated:

- Pain, burning, and tingling are treated with over-the-counter and prescription medication such as nonsteroidal anti-inflammatory drugs (NSAIDs), topical creams, COX-2 inhibitors, antidepressants, anticonvulsants, and opioids. [Gail again, as CKD patients we're out on the NSAIDS.]

- Numbness or complete loss of sensation can lead to complications such as ulcers, sores, and limb amputations. It is addressed by monitoring the affected areas — often the feet — for injuries and addressing wounds before they become more serious, as well as prescribing protective footwear and braces.

- Orthostatic hypotension (a drop in blood pressure upon standing up), which is an autonomic symptom, can be treated with increased sodium intake, a vasopressor such as ProAmatine (midodrine) to constrict blood vessels, a synthetic mineralocorticoid such as fludrocortisone to help maintain the balance of salt in the body, or a cholinesterase inhibitor such as pyridostigmine, which affects neurotransmitters.

- Gastroparesis, a delayed emptying of the stomach, is another autonomic symptom, which can be treated with medication to control nausea and vomiting, such as Reglan (metoclopramide), Ery-Tab (erythromycin), antiemetics, and antidepressants, as well as pain medication for abdominal discomfort.

- Motor neuropathy symptoms can include weakness and muscle wasting, particularly in the lower extremities, as well as deformities of the feet and loss of the Achilles' heel tendon reflex. Treatments can include physical therapy to regain strength, as well as braces and orthotics.

I've got to think about this. Any questions?

## 7/1/19  *Will B12 and Alpha Lipoic Acid Get Me Back to Dancing Sooner?*

Last week I wrote about diabetic neuropathy... and received quite a few comments from readers and the various communities I belong to. All were about B12 and/or Alpha Lipoic Acid. One person even commented about the veracity of articles about these two and he's right; science is constantly discovering new information that may contradict what we think we already know.

For now, I'm going to stick to what we think we already know. My experience was that I took Alpha Lipoic Acid for years and barely felt the neuropathy. Whoops! There I go again, plunging right in. Okay, time to back up.

Does anyone remember what neuropathy is? Young lady in the back of the room, thank you for raising your hand. According to The Foundation for Peripheral Neuropathy,

"There are many causes of peripheral neuropathy, including diabetes, chemo-induced neuropathy, hereditary disorders, inflammatory infections, auto-immune diseases, protein abnormalities, exposure to toxic chemicals (toxic neuropathy), poor nutrition, kidney failure, chronic alcoholism, and certain medications – especially those used to treat cancer and HIV/AIDS. In some cases, however, even with extensive evaluation, the causes of peripheral neuropathy in some people remain unknown – this is called idiopathic neuropathy."

Hmmm, that deals more with the causes. Let's try again. Sweetheart? (My husband has a question.) Yes, I wondered about the term 'peripheral,' too. I don't really know, but WebMD does:

## What Is Peripheral Neuropathy?

The name of the condition tells you a bit about what it is:

Peripheral: Beyond (in this case, beyond the brain and the spinal cord.)
Neuro-: Related to the nerves
-pathy: Disease

Peripheral neuropathy refers to the conditions that result when nerves that carry messages to and from the brain and spinal cord from and to the rest of the body are damaged or diseased.

The peripheral nerves make up an intricate network that connects the brain and spinal cord to the muscles, skin, and internal organs. Peripheral nerves come out of the spinal cord and are arranged along lines in the body called dermatomes. Typically, damage to a nerve will affect one or more dermatomes, which can be tracked to specific areas of the body. Damage to these nerves interrupts communication between the brain and other parts of the body and can impair muscle movement, prevent normal sensation in the arms and legs, and cause pain."

Oh, I think I understand better why I had a brain scan last week. I have the results, but need help interpreting them. Good thing I have an appointment at the Research Institute tomorrow.

I don't know about you, but I'm learning a lot from today's blog. Hold on, my neighbor has a question about what Alpha Lipoic Acid is supposed to do for peripheral neuropathy in the first place. Let's find out. Here's what MedicalNewsToday has to say:

"Alpha-lipoic acid is an organic compound in the body that acts as a potent antioxidant. It may have several health benefits.

While the body produces alpha-lipoic acid (ALA) naturally, a person can boost their levels by making suitable dietary choices, taking supplements, or both.

Supplementing with ALA is becoming increasingly popular, as some people believe that it may help with weight loss, diabetes, memory loss, skin health, and other health conditions.

In this article, learn about its effectiveness, possible benefits, and side effects.

**What is ALA?**

People can increase their ALA levels by taking supplements.

ALA is present within mitochondria, which are the powerhouses of the cells.

ALA is crucial for digestion, absorption, and the creation of energy. It helps enzymes turn nutrients into energy. It also has antioxidant properties.

Since humans can only produce ALA in small amounts, many people turn to supplements to increase their intake.

And now I know why I cannot take it. As a person being treated for pancreatic cancer (or any kind of cancer you may be treated for), antioxidants are the last thing I want to put in my body. I'll explain, Cuz.

OncologyNutrition.Org offers this information. Mind you, this is only part of what I read on this site.

"...some studies indicate that taking antioxidant supplements may interfere with chemotherapy and radiation therapy, by reducing their effectiveness. It is possible that antioxidants may protect tumor cells, in addition to healthy cells, from the oxidative damage intentionally caused by conventional treatments. This, in turn, may reduce the effectiveness of the treatments ...."

Too bad for me. Well, maybe B12??? Thanks for suggesting the MayoClinic, daughter. We'll look at it right now. I'm comfortable with the MayoClinic's information.

"The jury is still out on whether or not taking vitamin B-12 supplements can help treat diabetic neuropathy. Some small studies have shown a lessening of pain and other abnormal sensations. But, recent reviews of all of the research suggest that there's no significant benefit in taking B-12 supplements for diabetic neuropathy for people without a deficiency of the vitamin."

My labs have never shown any vitamin B deficiencies, but I think it may be more important to find out if B12 affects chemotherapy or radiation... or vice versa. I stumbled across this information during my search. It's from CancerResearchUK.org.

"Some dietary supplements can cause skin sensitivity and severe reactions when taken during radiotherapy treatment.

Some vitamins or minerals could interfere with how well cancer drugs work. Antioxidant supplements such as co enzyme Q10, selenium and the vitamins A, C and E can help to prevent cell damage. So some doctors think this might stop chemotherapy working well.

Get advice from your doctor, specialist, nurse, or dietitian if you want to take supplements and are having any kind of cancer treatment."

Notice B12 is not an antioxidant, but considering I'll be starting radiation (another term for radiotherapy) this week, I would like to avoid the possibility of either a 'severe reaction' or 'skin sensitivity.'

Looks like both Alpha Lipoic Acid and B12 are out for me as a cancer patient. Do talk to your doctor about both if you are not a cancer patient and are experiencing peripheral neuropathy. Thank you all for participating in this inquiry.

## 7/8/19 *Platelets, Blood, and RSNHope or a Little Bit of This and a Little Bit of That*

A reader from India asked me why I kept writing about chemotherapy. I explained that I have pancreatic cancer and that was part of my treatment. Chronic Kidney Disease patients may develop kidney cancer, although this type of cancer is not restricted to CKD patients. They also may develop another type of cancer that has nothing to do with the kidneys. Everyone's experience with chemotherapy is different, but I thought one person's experience was better than none. Here's hoping you *never* have to deal with any kind of cancer or chemotherapy, however.

While we're on explanations, I have a correction to make. The nurses at the Pancreatic Cancer Research Institute here in Arizona are a fount of knowledge. One of them heard me talking to my daughter about a platelet infusion and corrected me. It seems it's a platelet transfusion, just as it's a blood transfusion.

According to The Free Medical Dictionary

"in·fu·sion

(in-fyū'zhŭn),

1. The process of steeping a substance in water, either cold or hot (below the boiling point), to extract its soluble principles.

2. A medicinal preparation obtained by steeping the crude drug in water.

3. The introduction of fluid other than blood, for example, saline solution, into a vein."

The same dictionary, tells us:

"Transfusion is the process of transferring whole blood or blood components from one person (donor) to another (recipient)."

Therein lays the difference. Platelets are part of the blood, so it's a platelet transfusion. I'm glad that's straightened out.

While we're on this topic, here's a chart of compatible blood types for transfusions… always a handy thing to have.

| Blood Type of Recipient | Preferred Blood Type of Donor | If Preferred Blood Type Unavailable, Permissible Blood Type of Donor |
|---|---|---|
| A | A | O |
| B | B | O |
| AB | AB | A, B, O |
| O | O | No alternate types |

O is the universal blood type and, as you've probably noticed, is compatible with all blood types. The plus or minus sign after your blood type refers to being RH negative or positive. For example, my blood type is B+. That means I have type B blood and am RH positive.

I've had platelet transfusions several times since I was leaking blood here and there. Nothing like eating lunch and having nasal blood drip into your salad. Ugh! You also become weak and your hemoglobin goes down. Not a good situation at all. You know I'm hoping you never need one, but who knows what can happen in the future. Just in case you've forgotten what platelets are, Macmillan Cancer Support is here to help us out.

"Platelets are tiny cells in your blood which form clots to help stop bleeding. They develop from stem cells in the bone marrow (the spongy material inside the bones). They are then released from your bone marrow into your blood and travel around your body in your bloodstream. Platelets usually survive for 7–10 days before being destroyed naturally in your body or being used to clot the blood."

You'll probably notice the term "RH Positive" (unless you're RH Negative, of course) written on the platelet transfusion bag. You know I had to find out why. Memorial Sloan Cancer Center offers this information about your blood that will help us understand:

"Your blood type is either A, B, AB, or O. It's either Rh positive (+) or Rh negative (-).

Your blood type is checked with a test called a type and cross-match. The results of this test are used to match your blood type with the blood in our blood bank. Your healthcare provider will check to make sure that the blood is the correct match for you before they give you the transfusion."

The MayoClinic clarifies just what Rh Positive means:

"Rhesus (Rh) factor is an inherited protein found on the surface of red blood cells. If your blood has the protein, you're Rh positive. If your blood lacks the protein, you're Rh negative.

Rh positive is the most common blood type. Having an Rh negative blood type is not an illness and usually does not affect your health. However, it can affect your pregnancy. "

What I found especially interesting is that,

"If you have Rh-positive blood, you can get Rh-positive or Rh-negative blood. But if you have Rh-negative blood, you should only get Rh-negative blood. Rh-negative blood is used for emergencies when there's no time to test a person's Rh type."

Thank you to Health Jade for this information. This is a new site for me. You might want to take a look since their illustrations make so much clear.

Switching topics now. Are you aware of the Renal Support Network? Lori Hartwell is one of the most active CKD and dialysis people I've met in the entire nine years I've been writing about CKD. For example, she has this wonderful salad bar help for the renal diet:

"Choose: lettuce escarole, endive, alfalfa sprouts, celery sticks, cole slaw, cauliflower, cucumbers, green beans, green peas, green peppers, radishes, zucchini, better, eggs (chopped), tuna in spring water, parmesan cheese, Chinese noodles, gelatin salads, Italian low calorie dressing, vinaigrette, low fat dressing.

Avoid: avocado, olives, raisins, tomatoes, pickles, bacon bits, chickpeas, kidney beans nuts, shredded cheddar cheese, three bean salads, sunflower seeds, Chow Mein noodles, fried bread croutons, potato salad, thick salad dressing, relishes"

What could be easier than printing this out and sticking it in your wallet? But Lori is not just about the renal diet. She also posts CKD

& dialysis podcasts at KidneyTalk 24/7 Podcast Radio Show. All this and more are on the website. I must admit I look forward to the RSNHope magazine each quarter.

## 7/15/19 *Not Nuked*

Friday, I saw my oncology radiologist after having had a week of radiation treatments. As he was explaining what the radiation was meant to do to the remaining third of the tumor and how it was being done, one sentence he uttered stood out to me: "This doesn't work like your microwave."

Since radiation is also used in treating kidney cancer… and any other kind of cancer, to the best of my knowledge… I decided to take a look at that statement. First we need to know how a microwave works, so we know how radiation treatment for cancer *doesn't* work. I went to the Health Sciences Academy for an explanation.

"How do microwaves work?

Before we talk about how microwaves heat your food, let's make a distinction between two very different kinds of radiation:

1. ionising radiation, and

2. non-ionising radiation.

Ionising radiation, which can remove tightly-bound electrons from atoms, causing them to become charged, is less risky in very tiny amounts (such as x-rays) but can cause problems when exposure is high (think burns and even DNA damage). However, microwaves emit non-ionising radiation; a type of radiation that has enough energy to move atoms around within a molecule but not enough to remove electrons.

What does this mean? Because the radiation from microwaves is non-ionising, it can only cause molecules in the food to move. …

In other words, microwave radiation cannot alter the chemical structure of food components. More precisely, when heating food in a microwave, the radiation that the microwave produces is actually absorbed by the water molecules in the food. This energy causes the water molecules to vibrate, generating heat through this (harmless) friction, which cooks the food. This mechanism is what makes microwaves much faster at heating food than other methods. Its energy immediately reaches molecules that are about an inch below the outer surface of the food, whereas heat from other cooking methods moves into food gradually via conduction...."

Phew, I'm glad to know I'm not being cooked from the inside. But what is happening to me and everyone else who has radiation as a cancer treatment? I went straight to the American Cancer Society for the answer.

"Radiation therapy uses high-energy particles or waves, such as x-rays, [Gail here: this is ionising radiation.] gamma rays, electron beams, or protons, to destroy or damage cancer cells.

Your cells normally grow and divide to form new cells. But cancer cells grow and divide faster than most normal cells. Radiation works by making small breaks in the DNA inside cells. These breaks keep cancer cells from growing and dividing and cause them to die. Nearby normal cells can also be affected by radiation, but most recover and go back to working the way they should.

Unlike chemotherapy, which usually exposes the whole body to cancer-fighting drugs, radiation therapy is usually a local treatment. In most cases, it's aimed at and affects only the part of the body being treated. Radiation treatment is planned to damage cancer cells, with as little harm as possible to nearby healthy cells.

Some radiation treatments (systemic radiation therapy) use radioactive substances that are given in a vein or by mouth. Even though this type of radiation does travel throughout the body, the radioactive substance mostly collects in the area of the tumor, so there's little effect on the rest of the body."

I don't know how many times this was explained to me, but seeing it now in black and white suddenly makes it clear. So this means I've had four months of my entire body being attacked – in a lifesaving way, of course – now only the cancer cells are being attacked.

Yet, I am experiencing some side effects even after only one week of radiation. I wondered if that's usual. Cancer.net answered that question for me.

"Why does radiation therapy cause side effects?

High doses of radiation therapy are used to destroy cancer cells. Side effects come from damage to healthy cells and tissues near the treatment area. Major advances in radiation therapy have made it more precise. This reduces the side effects.

Some people experience few side effects from radiation therapy. Or even none. Other people experience more severe side effects.

Reactions to the radiation therapy often start during the second or third week of treatment. They may last for several weeks after the final treatment.

Are there options to prevent or treat these side effects?

Yes. Your health care team can help you prevent or treat many side effects. Preventing and treating side effects is an important part of cancer treatment. This is called palliative care or supportive care.

**Potential side effects**

Radiation therapy is a local treatment. This means that it only affects the area of the body where the tumor is located. For example, people do not usually lose their hair from having radiation therapy. But radiation therapy to the scalp may cause hair loss.

Common side effects of radiation therapy include:

**Skin problems.** Some people who receive radiation therapy experience dryness, itching, blistering, or peeling. These side effects depend on which part of the body received radiation therapy. Skin problems usually go away a few weeks after treatment ends. If skin damage becomes a serious problem, your doctor may change your treatment plan.

**Fatigue.** Fatigue describes feeling tired or exhausted almost all the time. Your level of fatigue often depends on your treatment plan. For example, radiation therapy combined with chemotherapy may result in more fatigue….

**Long-term side effects.** Most side effects go away after treatment. But some continue, come back, or develop later. These are called late effects. One example is the development of a second cancer. This is a new type of cancer that develops because of the original cancer treatment. The risk of this late effect is low. And the risk is often smaller than the benefit of treating the primary, existing cancer."

Funny how I managed to forget about late effects, even though my oncology team made it clear this could happen. I think having the radiation to rid myself of *this* cancer is worth the risk.

## 7/22/19 *What's That Got to Do with My Occupation?*

I've written about neuropathy, but what is this occupational therapy that may treat it? I know about physical therapy and have made use of it when necessary. Remember a few years ago when knee surgery was indicated? Physical therapy helped me avoid the surgery.

This time I was offered gabapentin for the neuropathy. That's a drug usually used for epilepsy which can also help with neuropathy. I would explain how it works, but no one seems to know. I had two problems with this drug:

1. Gabapentin became a controlled substance in England as of April of this year. England always seem to be one step ahead of the U.S. re medications.

2. It is not suggested if you have kidney disease.

My other option was occupational therapy. That's the one I chose. Let's backtrack a bit for a definition of occupational therapy. Thank you to my old buddy (since college over 50 years ago) the Merriam-Webster Dictionary for the following definition.

"therapy based on engagement in meaningful activities of daily life (such as self-care skills, education, work, or social interaction) especially to enable or encourage participation in such activities despite impairments or limitations in physical or mental functioning"

That got me to wondering just how occupational therapy differed from physical therapy, the kind of therapy with which I was already familiar. I went to my old buddy again for any hints I could pick up from the definition for physical therapy.

"therapy for the preservation, enhancement, or restoration of movement and physical function impaired or threatened by disease, injury, or disability that utilizes therapeutic exercise, physical modalities (such as massage and electrotherapy), assistive devices, and patient education and training"

Made sense to me. Physical therapy was for the movement of the body, while occupational therapy was to help you carry out the tasks of your daily life. For example, it takes me longer to write a blog because my tingling, yet numb, fingers often slip into the spaces between the keys on the keyboard. Another example is that I now use a cane since I can't tell if my tingling, yet numb, feet are flat on the floor as I walk.

Something I found interesting about occupational therapy is that it uses many forms of therapy that were once considered alternative medicine… like electrical energy. What's that you say? You'd like an example?

Well, here you go. My therapist uses a machine called a Havimat. The following is from the National Stem Cell Institute and explains what the Havimat can do and how.

"….The therapist connects an electronic lead to his/her wrist while the patient grasps a small cylinder grip. The vinyl gloves that the therapist wears prevents the circuit of electric current from closing, thus creating the 'push-pull' effect that penetrates deeply into tissues. Meanwhile, the patient's experience is one of a pleasant, deep massage maintained by the therapist's gentle pressure as he/she directs the deep oscillation.

…. The therapy 'un-dams' trapped fluid. Tissues are decongested and edema is significantly reduced. This shrinks swelling in the area being treated. Hivamat has been shown to be exceptionally effective in relieving lymphedema when used by therapists to enhance manual lymphatic drainage.

…. Besides the reduction of edema, therapists use Hivamat for ridding tissues of toxins [Gail here: like chemotherapy.] When used by a certified therapist during a manipulation technique known as manual lymphatic drainage, the therapy improves lymph fluid movement. This encourages better flow through the lymphatic system, which then carries away metabolic waste and toxins more quickly. Hivamat also promotes the production of lymphocytes, which improve the function of the immune system. [Gail again: as CKD patients, our immune systems are compromised.]"

There is one thing, though. Apparently, the Havimat is NOT suggested if there is an active tumor. Uh-oh, I had three treatments with the Havimat before I uncovered that fact. I'll have to speak with my therapist today and find out why she didn't know that. But it is clear that using electrical energy as treatment is another case of what was formerly considered alternative medicine becoming mainstream medicine.

Topic switch. I've written about the American Association of Kidney Patients (AAKP), precision care, and clinical trials many times before. You're probably already aware of the new initiative for patient care. AAKP wants your help in doing their part as far as patient experience with this survey.

"As part of AAKP's National Strategy, we have expanded our

capacities to involve a far larger, and more representative, number of patients in research opportunities and clinical trials. The results of these research opportunities and clinical trials will help create a clearer understanding of the patient experience and help shape the future of kidney disease treatment and care. *AAKP is fully committed to changing the status quo of kidney care and to better aligning treatment to personal aspirations.*

To achieve this goal, the AAKP Center for Patient Research & Education is working with top researchers to ensure that the patient voice, patient preferences and patient perceptions are heard.

AAKP is very pleased to partner with *Northwestern University* and *University of Pennsylvania* on an important research project organ donation.

Please consider taking part in this online survey and help shape the future of kidney care for you and those yet to be diagnosed.

## 7/29/19 *But Why?*

As Chronic Kidney Disease patients, we all know that proteinuria is one indication of our disease. Would you like a reminder about what proteinuria is? Here's one from The American Kidney Fund:

"Healthy kidneys remove extra fluid and waste from your blood, but let proteins and other important nutrients pass through and return to your blood stream. When your kidneys are not working as well as they should, they can let some protein (albumin) escape through their filters, into your urine. When you have protein in your urine, it is called proteinuria (or albuminuria). Having protein in your urine can be a sign of nephrotic syndrome, or an early sign of kidney disease."

I used to think that's all it was: an indicator of CKD. That is until my occupational therapist and I got to talking about the edema caused by neuropathy.

Ah! Flash! We did also talk about Havimat which I wrote about last week and I checked on a number of sites to see if it were safe for an active tumor. The consensus of the sites agreed it was safe to use on someone with an active tumor that was being treated as long as it was not used on the location of the tumor itself. I feel better now about having had three sessions with Havimat since the occupational therapist was careful not to use it anywhere near my pancreas – the site of the tumor.

But I digress. Back to the topic at hand: proteinuria. It seems that protein is needed in the body, rather than being excreted in the urine. You guessed it. My question became the topic of today's blog: But Why?

According to WebMD:

"Protein is an important component of every cell in the body. Hair and nails are mostly made of protein. Your body uses protein to build and repair tissues. You also use protein to make enzymes, hormones, and other body chemicals. Protein is an important building block of bones, muscles, cartilage, skin, and blood."

Okay, got it that protein is very necessary but what does that have to do with the chemotherapy I had that seemed to cause the proteinuria problem? After looking at bunches of different sites (Today's blog is taking a very long time to write.), I gleaned a little hint here and a little hint there until I figured out that certain types of chemotherapy may make proteinuria worse if you already have it, or cause it. Boo for me; I lost on that one since I already had proteinuria.

Well, what about the edema from the neuropathy? Was proteinuria affecting that in some way? Or did I have it backwards and it was the neuropathy that was causing the edema. I went to eMedicineHealth for some help with this.

"Certain drugs and medications can cause nerve damage. Examples include cancer therapy drugs such as vincristine (Oncovin, Vincasar), and antibiotics such as metronidazole (Flagyl), and isoniazid (Nydrazid, Laniazid)."

This little tidbit is from MedicalNewsToday:

"Chemotherapy can damage nerves that affect feeling and movement in the hands and feet. Doctors call this condition chemotherapy-induced peripheral neuropathy (CIPN). Symptoms can be severe and may affect a person's quality of life."

By the way, diabetic neuropathy is another form of peripheral neuropathy.

The HonorHealth Research Institute in Scottsdale, Arizona, where I'm being treated offered both the gabapentin for the pain (which I skipped since I want to try non-drug treatment first) and occupational therapy. Let's see what that might do for me. Please note that occupational therapy works at reducing the pain of the neuropathy.

I have a bag of toys. Each has a different sensory delivery on my hands and feet. For example, there's a woven metal ring that I run up and down my fingers and toes, then up my arms and legs. I do the same with most of the other toys: a ball with netting over it, another with rubber strings hanging from it. I also have a box of uncooked rice to rub my feet and hands in… and lots of other toys. The idea is to desensitize my hands and feet.

I was also given physical exercises to do, like raising my fisted hands above my head and straightening out my fist several times. This is one of many exercises. Do you remember the old TV show, *E.R*? It takes me slightly longer than one 43 minute episode to complete the exercises.

The therapist uses the Havimat (electrical stimulation), another machine that sucks the chemo out, and a third that pulses. I am amazed at how the edema disappears when she uses these. The effect doesn't stay very long. Compression socks have helped and, despite their not-so-pleasing appearance are quite comfortable.

Proteinuria *is* so much more than just an indication that you may have Chronic Kidney Disease.

## 8/5/19 *Which Comes First?*

Periodically, a blog will actually be the response to a reader's question. I've received several questions lately. The first thing I do when I receive a question is to be sure the reader understands that I am not a doctor and that no matter what I research for them, they must clear the information with their nephrologist before taking any action. Today's question was asked by a long time reader who already understands my terms for researching for her.

That's a pretty big build up for a common sense question. But, at least now you understand how I handle reader questions and may want to ask one (or more) of your own.

Back to the question at hand: What is the connection between PTH and creatinine and which causes a problem with the other?

What's PTH, you ask. Let's find out. You and your Hormones: an educational source from the Society of Endocrinology was a great deal of help here:

"Alternative names for parathyroid hormone

PTH; parathormone; parathyrin

What is parathyroid hormone?

The parathyroid glands are located in the neck, just behind the butterfly-shaped thyroid gland.

Parathyroid hormone is secreted from four parathyroid glands, which are small glands in the neck, located behind the thyroid gland. Parathyroid hormone regulates calcium levels in the blood, largely by increasing the levels when they are too low. It does this through its actions on the kidneys, bones and intestine:

1. Bones – parathyroid hormone stimulates the release of calcium from large calcium stores in the bones into the bloodstream. This increases bone destruction and decreases the formation of new bone.

2. Kidneys – parathyroid hormone reduces loss of calcium in urine. Parathyroid hormone also stimulates the production of active vitamin D in the kidneys.

3. Intestine – parathyroid hormone indirectly increases calcium absorption from food in the intestine, via its effects on vitamin D metabolism"

Got it? Okay then let's remind ourselves what creatinine is. I wrote the following in last December 24$^{th}$'s blog:

"A good place to start is always at the beginning. By this, I wonder if I mean the beginning of my Chronic Kidney Disease awareness advocacy as the author of **What Is It and How Did I Get It? Early Stage Chronic Kidney Disease** and the blog *or* if I mean the basics about creatinine. Let's combine them all. The following definition is from the book which became the earliest blogs:

'**Creatinine clearance**: Compares the creatinine level in your urine with that in your blood to provide information about your kidney function'

Hmmm, that didn't exactly work. Let's try again. Bingo! It was in ***SlowItDownCKD 2014,***

'Creatinine: chemical waste product that's produced by our muscle metabolism and to a smaller extent by eating meat. {MayoClinic.org}'"

That was nine years ago, but the information remains the same today.

So now, we know what both PTH and creatinine are, but what's the connection? According to VIVO Pathophysiology, Colorado State University:

"**Suppression of calcium loss in urine**: In addition to stimulating fluxes of calcium into blood from bone and intestine, parathyroid hormone puts a brake on excretion of calcium in urine, thus conserving calcium in blood. This effect is mediated by stimulating tubular reabsorption of calcium. Another effect of parathyroid hormone on the kidney is to stimulate loss of phosphate ions in urine."

To recap so far, we know what both PTH and creatinine are and what the connection between the two is. Now we need to know if one causes the other and, if so, which.

"**Chronic kidney failure.** Your kidneys convert vitamin D into a form that your body can use. If your kidneys function poorly, usable vitamin D may decline and calcium levels drop. Chronic kidney failure is the most common cause of secondary hyperparathyroidism."

Thank you to the Mayo Clinic for this information.

Whoops! You may need a few reminders to understand the Mayo Clinic's information, so here they are. Vitamin D helps the body absorb calcium properly. Calcium is necessary for strong bones and teeth. Many people don't know it's also necessary for blood clotting, nerves and heart. 'Hyper' means over or, in this case, high as in above the necessary. Remember that when calcium or vitamin D is low, PTH rises. In my mind's eye, I see a scale balancing the two out.

I did not find any information about PTH causing high creatinine. That doesn't mean there isn't any. It just means there isn't any I could access. I found a journal site that looked promising, but it turned out to be for endocrinologists only. Too bad for us.

I do hope I've answered my reader's question to her satisfaction. I know I enjoyed learning all this new information.

## 8/12/19 *That Looks Swollen*

Remember I mentioned that several readers have asked questions that would become blogs? For example, one reader's question became last week's blog concerning creatinine and PTH. Another reader's question became this week's blog about lymphedema. She was diagnosed with it and wondered if it had anything to do with her protein buildup.

She's a long time reader and online friend, so she already knows I remind those that ask questions that I am not a doctor and, no matter what I discover, she must speak with her nephrologist before taking any action based on what I wrote. That is always true.

I'm a CKD patient just like you. The only difference is that I know how to research (Teaching college level Research Writing taught me a lot.) and happen to have been a writer for decades before I was diagnosed. Just take a look at my Amazon Author Page. But enough about me.

Anyone know what lymphedema is? I didn't when I first heard the word, although my Hunter College of C.U.N.Y education as an English teacher gave me some clues. Edema had something to do with swelling under the skin. Actually, we can get more specific with The Free Medical Dictionary:

"suffix meaning swelling resulting from an excessive accumulation of serious fluid in the tissues of the body in (specified) locations"

I took a guess that lymph had to do with the lymph nodes. Using the same dictionary, I found this:

"The almost colourless fluid that bathes body tissues and is found in the lymphatic vessels that drain the tissues of the fluid that fil ters across the blood vessel walls from blood. Lymph carries antibodies and lymphocytes (white blood cells that help fight infection) that have entered the lymph nodes from the blood."

Time to attach the suffix (group of letters added at the end of a word that changes its meaning) to the root (most basic meaning of the word) to come up with a definition of lymphedema. No, not my definition, the same dictionary's.

"Swelling, especially in subcutaneous tissues, as a result of obstruction of lymphatic vessels or lymph nodes, with accumulation of lymph in the affected region."

Okay, we know what lymphedema is now but what – if anything – does that have to do with proteinuria? This is the closest I could come to an answer that

1. Wasn't too medical for me to understand and
2. Had anything to do with the kidneys.

"A thorough medical history and physical examination are done to rule out other causes of limb swelling, such as edema due to congestive heart failure, kidney failure, blood clots, or other conditions."

Thank you, MedicineNet.

My friend, while a Chronic Kidney Disease patient, is not in renal failure. Was there something I missed?

Johns Hopkins Medicine gives us our first clue. It seems that lymphedema is a buildup of a specific fluid: protein-rich,

"Lymphedema is an abnormal buildup of protein-rich fluid in any part of the body as a result of malfunction in the lymphatic system."

Malfunction in the lymphatic system? What could cause that? According to Lymphatic Education & Research:

"Secondary Lymphedema (acquired regional lymphatic insufficiency) is a disease that is common among adults and children in the United States. It can occur following any trauma, infection or surgery that disrupts the lymphatic channels or results in the loss of lymph nodes. Among the more than 3 million breast cancer survivors alone, acquired or secondary lymphedema is believed to be present in approximately 30% of these individuals, predisposing them to the same long-term problems as described above. Lymphedema also results from prostate, uterine, cervical, abdominal, orthopedic cosmetic (liposuction) and other surgeries, malignant melanoma, and treatments used for both Hodgkin's and non-Hodgkin's lymphoma. Radiation, sports injuries, tattooing, and any physical insult to the lymphatic pathways can also cause lymphedema. Even though lymphatic insufficiency may not immediately present at the time any of the events occur, these individuals are at life-long risk for the onset of lymphedema."

I know the reader who has asked the question has a complex medical history that may include one or more of the conditions listed above. As for the protein buildup, we already know that kidneys which are not working well don't filter the protein from your blood as well as they could. So, is there a connection between this reader's protein buildup and her lymphedema? Sure looks like it.

While the following is from BreastCancer.org, it is a simple explanation that may apply to other causes of lymphedema, too:

"… lymph nodes and vessels can't keep up with the tissues' need to get rid of extra fluid, **proteins** (Gail here: my bolding), and waste… the proteins and wastes do not get filtered out of the lymph as efficiently as they once did. Very gradually, waste and fluid buildup…. "

8/19/19 *Adult Toys*

In keeping with my promise to myself that August would be answer-readers'-questions month, this week I'll be writing about the occupational therapy toys a reader asked about. Did you think I meant the other kind of adult toys? Hmmm, maybe it would make sense to know why toys are used in dealing with neuropathy in the first place.

As my occupational therapist explained it, the therapy toys are used to stimulate the nerve endings to bud so that new pathways may be created. I don't fully understand it, but this is what I wrote in my July 29$^{th}$ blog:

"I have a bag of toys. Each has a different sensory delivery on my hands and feet. For example, there's a woven metal ring that I run up and down my fingers and toes, then up my arms and legs. I do the same with most of the other toys: a ball with netting over it, another with rubber strings hanging from it. I also have a box of uncooked rice to rub my feet and hands in… and lots of other toys. The idea is to desensitize my hands and feet."

Ah, but now we know these therapy toys are used for more. Desensitization? Good. Building new pathways for sensations? Better. Yes, I want my hands and feet to stop feeling so tingly all the time, but I also want to be able to feel whatever it is I'm holding or touching. Remember, for me, this was an unexpected side effect of chemotherapy, although it could have just as easily been diabetic peripheral neuropathy. Aha! Now you see why I've included this in the blog posts in the first place: Diabetes is the number one cause of Chronic Kidney Disease.

Ready to explore some therapy toys? Well, all rightee. Let's start with my favorite, the one I call the smoosh ball. Oh, since I bought a bag full of these different therapy toys on Amazon, none were labeled so I made up my own names for them. Hey, I'm a writer. I can get away with that.

This one is soft and rubbery. It's the "another with rubber strings hanging from it," mentioned above that I rub on my toes and up my legs, then my fingers and up my arms as I do with most of these therapy toys. It causes the loveliest goose bumps. I'm surprised that Shiloh, our 80 pound dog, doesn't go after it just for the way it seems to shimmer. I also squeeze the smoosh ball with each hand.

The opposite of the smoosh ball is the steel ring. This one is almost painful if I'm not careful. In addition to using it on my hands, arms, fingers, and toes as I did the smoosh ball, I also use it as a ring on each toe and finger moving it up and down. Notice I'm not mentioning how many repetitions I do for each of the therapy toys. That's because everyone is different. Your neuropathy may be worse than mine, or – hopefully – not as bad as mine.

The pea pod is the hardest therapy toy for me to use. The idea is to squeeze the pod to cause the peas to pop up one by one. Sounds easy, right? Nope. You need to isolate these fingers you can't even feel until you get the right ones pressing on the right places to make that little fellow pop out.

The brush is a comforting therapy toy. I wonder if this is why horses like being curried (brushed). It's a soft, rubber brush which feels almost luxuriant as I rub it up my fingers, arms, toes, and legs. It was also the first therapy toy I was introduced to since the occupational therapist used it during my first treatment.

Then there's the ball with the netting around it. I do the usual rub the fingers, arms, toes, and legs with it. I also squeeze it like a stress ball. It feels completely different than the smoosh ball and even makes a sort of flatulence sound when I squeeze it. Well, that was unexpected.

I have a small ball that looks like a globe. Maybe that's because children use these therapy toys, too? All I can figure out to do with this is to squeeze it like a stress ball. I'll have to remember to ask the occupational therapist if that's what it's meant for.

The little beads can defeat me. The idea is to place them in a bowl and then pick them up using your thumb and the different fingers one at a time. At first, I was using my long nails to pick them up. Once I realized what I was doing, I cut my nails. It is surprising to me to realize how weak some of my fingers are as compared to how strong others are.

The mesh has a bead in it. You move it back and forth from one end of the mesh to the other, using each finger plus your thumb individually. Of course, this one feels really good on the toes, legs, fingers, and arms because it's a soft mesh (but not as soft as the mesh on the net ball).

The snake is a long piece of soft rubber. Before I execute the usual rubbing on the toes, legs, fingers, and arms, I use it the way you use an elastic band for stretching across your chest. It is more flexible than you'd think.

Not part of my bag of tricks – I mean therapy toys – is the foot roller. This is another therapy toy I bought on Amazon after trying one out at an occupational therapy treatment. Have you ever heard the expression 'hurts so good?' That's what this feels like while you roll it back and forth under your feet. Lest you get me wrong, it does not hurt enough to make you want to stop, just enough to make those tingly feet tingle even more.

I also do stretching exercises for my hands, place my feet in rice, and try to pick up a wash cloth with my toes. It takes a long time to exercise, but I think it's worth it.

8/26/19 *Stay in the Blood, PLEASE*

Let's finish out this lazy, hazy summer month of August with another reader question. This one was quite straight forward:

"Any advice to slow down protein leaking into urine. Hard to build muscle when you keep excreting protein"

The condition of leaking protein into your urine is called proteinuria. That's almost self-explanatory. The root of the word actually says protein while the suffix (group of related letters added to the end of a word which changes its meaning) is defined as,

"**-uria**.

1. suffix **meaning** the "presence of a substance in the urine": ammoniuria, calciuria, enzymuria.

2. combining form **meaning** "(condition of) possessing urine": paruria, polyuria, pyuria.

Thank you to the Medical Dictionary for the definition of uria.

Okay, so we know that protein is leaking into the urine. Not good. Why? We need it in our blood, not excreted in our urine. The following is from a previous blog on proteinuria. I used the dropdown menu in "Topics" on the right side of the blog page at **gailraegarwood.wordpress.com** to find it or any other topic listed there. You can, too.

"According to WebMD:

'Protein is an important component of every cell in the body. Hair and nails are mostly made of protein. Your body uses protein to build and repair tissues. You also use protein to make enzymes, hormones, and other body chemicals. Protein is an important building block of bones, muscles, cartilage, skin, and blood.'"

Got it. Our reader is correct; it is hard to build muscle if you're "excreting protein." Now what? I usually stick to medical sites but this comment from Healthfully caught my eye.

"Continue monitoring how much protein your kidneys are spilling for several months. Since colds and infections can cause transient increases in protein, you will want at least several months of data."

As Chronic Kidney Disease patients, we usually have quarterly urine tests… or, at least, I do. My urine protein level is included. I did not know that colds and infections are a factor here. Let's say our reader did not have a cold or infection. What else could she do to slow down this loss of protein via her urine?

The American Kidney Fund suggests the following:

"If you have diabetes or high blood pressure, the first and second most common causes of kidney disease, it is important to make sure these conditions are under control.

If you have diabetes, controlling it will mean checking your blood sugar often, taking medicines as your doctor tells you to, and following a healthy eating and exercise plan. If you have high blood pressure, your doctor may tell you to take a medicine to help lower your blood pressure and protect your kidneys from further damage. The types of medicine that can help with blood pressure and proteinuria are called angiotensin-converting enzyme inhibitors (ACE inhibitors) and angiotensin receptor blockers (ARBs).

If you have protein in your urine, but you do not have diabetes or high blood pressure, an ACE inhibitor or an ARB may still help to protect your kidneys from further damage. If you have protein in your urine, talk to your doctor about choosing the best treatment option for you."

So far, we've discovered that frequent urine testing, determining if you have a cold or infection, keeping your diabetes and blood pressure under control, and/or ACE inhibitors may be helpful. But here's my eternal question: What else can slow down the spilling of protein into our urine?

The Kidney & Urology Foundation of America, Inc. has some more ideas about that:

"In addition to blood glucose and blood pressure control, restricting dietary salt and protein intake is recommended. Your doctor may refer you to a dietitian to help you develop and follow a healthy eating plan."

As CKD patients, we know we need to cut down on salt intake. I actually eliminate added salt and have banned the salt shakers from the kitchen. No wonder no one but me likes my cooking. You do lose your taste for salt eventually. After all these years, I taste salt in restaurant food that makes that particular food unpalatable to me.

Hmmm, it seems to me that a list of high protein foods might be helpful here.

POULTRY…

- **Skinless chicken breast** – 4oz – 183 Calories – 30g Protein – 0 Carbs – 7g Fat

- **Skinless chicken (Dark)** – 4 oz – 230 Calories – 32g Protein – 0 Carbs – 5g Fat

- **Skinless Turkey (White)** – 4 oz – 176 Calories – 34g Protein – 0 Carbs – 3.5g Fat

- **Skinless Turkey (Dark)** – 4 oz – 211 Calories – 31g Protein – 0 Carbs – 8.1 g Fat

FISH…

- **Salmon** – 3 oz – 119 Calories – 17g Protein – 0 Carbs – 5.5g Fat

- **Halibut** – 3 oz – 91 Calories – 18g Protein – 0 Carbs – 3g Fat

- **Tuna** – 1/4 cup – 70 Calories – 18g Protein – 0 Carbs – 0g Fat

- **Mackerel** – 3 oz – 178 Calories – 16.1g Protein – 0 Carbs – 12g Fat

- **Anchovies** (packed in water) – 1 oz – 42 Calories – 6g Protein – 1.3g Fat

- **Flounder** – 1 127g fillet – 149 Calories – 30.7g Protein – 0 Carbs – 0.5g Fat (High Cholesterol)

- **Swordfish** – 1 piece 106g – 164 Calories – 26.9g Protein – 0 Carbs – 1.5g Fat (High Cholesterol)

- **Cod** – 1 fillet 180g – 189 Calories – 41.4g protein – 0 Carbs – 0.3g Fat (High Cholesterol)

- **Herring** – 1 fillet 143g – 290 Calories – 32.9g Protein – 0 Carbs – 3.7g Fat (High Cholesterol)

- **Haddock** – 1 fillet 150g – 168 Calories – 36.4g Protein – 0 Carbs – 0.3g Fat (High Cholesterol)

- **Grouper** – fillet 202g – 238 Calories – 50.2g Protein – 0 Carbs – 0.6g Fat (High Cholesterol)

- **Snapper** – 1 fillet 170g – 218 Calories – 44.7g Protein – 0 Carbs – 0.6g Fat (High Cholesterol)

BEEF...

- **Eye of round steak** – 3 oz – 276 Calories – 49g Protein – 2.4g Fat

- **Sirloin tip side steak** – 3 oz -206 Calories – 39g Protein – 2g Fat

- **Top sirloin** – 3 oz – 319 Calories – 50.9g Protein – 4g Fat

- **Bottom round steak** – 3 oz – 300 Calories – 47g Protein – 3.5g Fat

- **Top round steak** – 3 oz – 240 Calories – 37g Protein – 3.1g Fat

PORK...

- **Pork loin** – 3 oz – 180 Calories – 25g Protein – 0 Carbs – 2.9g Fat (High in cholesterol)

- **Tenderloin**– 3 oz – 103 Calories – 18g Protein – 0.3g Carbs – 1.2g Fat (High in cholesterol)

GAME MEATS...

- **Bison** – 3 0z – 152 Calories – 21.6g Protein – 0 Carbs – 3g Fat

- **Rabbit** – 3 oz – 167 Calories – 24.7g Protein – 0 Carbs – 2.0g Fat

- **Venison** (Deer loin broiled) – 3 oz – 128 Calories – 25.7g Protein – 0 Carbs – 0.7g Fat

GRAINS...

- **Cooked Quinoa** – 1/2 cup – 115 Calories – 4.1g Protein – 22 Carbs – 2g Fat

- **Cooked Brown Rice** – 1/2 cup – 106 Calories – 2.7g Protein – 23 Carbs – 0.7g Fat

- **Regular Popcorn** (Air Popped no oil) – 1 cup – 60 Calories – 2g Protein – 11 Carbs – 0.6g Fat

- **Steel cut Oatmeal** – 1 cup – 145 Calories – 7g Protein – 25g Carbs – 2.5g Fat

- **Multi grain bread** – 1 slice – 68.9 Calories – 3.5g Protein – 11.3g Carbs – 0.2g Fat

BEANS (All nutrition values calculated for cooked beans)...

- **Tofu** – 1/2 cup – 98 Calories – 11g Protein – 2g Carbs – 6g Fat

- **Lentils** – 1/2 cup – 119 Calories – 9g Protein – 20g Carbs – 0.3g Fat

- **'Black beans** – 1/2 cup – 115 Calories – 7.8g Protein – 20 Carbs – 0.4g Fat

- **Kidney beans** – 1/2 cup – 111 Calories – 7.2g Protein – 20.2 Carbs – 0.4g Fat

- **Lima beans** – 1/2 cup – 110 Calories – 7.4g Protein – 19.7 Carbs – 0.3g Fat

- **Soy beans** – 1/2 cup – 133 Calories – 11g Protein – 10 Carbs – 5.9g Fat

DAIRY…

- **Skim milk** – 1 cup – 90 Calories – 9g Protein – 12g Carbs – 4.8g Fat

- **Low fat Yogurt** – 1 cup – 148 Calories – 12g Protein – 17Carbs – 3.2g Fat

- **Non fat Yogurt** – 1 cup – 130 Calories – 13g Protein – 16.9 Carbs – 0.4 Fat

- **Cheddar cheese** – 1 oz – 116 Calories – 7g Protein – 0.4 Carbs – 9.2g Fat

- **Low fat Cottage Cheese** – 1/2 cup – 82 Calories – 14g Protein – 3.1g Carbs – 0.7g Fat

- **One large egg** – 73 Calories – 6.6g Protein – 0 Carbs – 6g Fat

- **Low fat Milk** – 1 cup – 119 Calories – 8g Protein – 12 Carbs – 4.6g Fat

NUTS & SEEDS...

- **Raw Almonds** – 1 oz about 22 whole – 169 Calories – 22g Carbs – 6.2g Protein – 1.1g Fat

- **Raw Pistachios** – 1 oz about 49 Kernels – 157 Calories – 7.9g Carbs – 5.8g Protein – 1.5g Fat

- **Pumpkin seeds** – 1 oz – 28g about 100 hulled seeds – 151 Calories – 5g Carbs – 6.0g Protein – 2.4g Fat

- **Raw Macadamia nuts** – 1 oz about 10- 12 kernels – 203 Calories – 4g Carbs – 2.2g Protein – 3.4g Fat

- **Chia seeds** – 1 oz – 137 Calories – 12.3g Carbs – 4.4g Protein – 0.9g Fat

- **Walnuts** – 1 cup in shell about 7 total – 183 Calories – 3.8g Carbs – 4.3g Protein – 1.7g Fat

- **Raw Cashews** - 1 oz – 28g – 155 Calories – 9.2g Carbs – 5.1g Protein – 2.2g Fat

MORE HIGH PROTEIN FOODS...

- **Natural peanut butter** – 1 oz – 146 Calories – 7.3g Protein – 10g Carbs – 1.6g Fat

- **Natural almond butter** – 1 tbsp – 101 Calories – 2.4g Protein – 3.4 Carbs – 0.9g Fat

- **Natural cashew butter** – 1 tbsp – 93.9 Calories – 2.8g Protein – 4.4 Carbs – 1.6g Fat

- **Hummus** – 1 oz – 46.5 Calories – 2.2g Protein – 4.0g Carbs – 0.4g Fat

- **Tempeh Cooked** – 1 oz – 54 Calories – 5.1g Protein – 2.6g Carbs – 1.0g Fat

Be leery of protein sources that are not on your kidney diet.

## 9/2/19  How Will They Know?

Let's start this month with a guest blog by American Medical Alert IDs. Why? Although I am not endorsing this particular brand, because I clearly remember being give Sulphur drugs in the Emergency Room when I was by myself and unable to let the medical staff there know I have Chronic Kidney Disease. Why? Because I remember that my husband fell when I was out of town. His grown children took him to the emergency room but didn't know about his latex allergy and he was in no condition to explain.

### Everything You Need To Know About Medical Alert IDs for Chronic Kidney Disease

Are you debating on getting a medical alert ID for chronic kidney disease? It's time to take the confusion out of choosing and engraving a medical ID. This post will show you everything you need to know so you can enjoy the benefits of wearing one.

### Why Kidney Patients Should Wear a Medical Alert ID

A medical ID serves as an effective tool to alert emergency staff of a patient's special care needs, even when a person can't speak for themselves. When every second counts, wearing a medical ID can help protect the kidney and safeguard its remaining function.

In emergencies, anyone diagnosed with chronic kidney disease or kidney failure may require special medical attention and monitoring. It is important that patients are able to communicate and identify their medical condition at all times. This includes individuals who are:

- Undergoing in-center hemodialysis

- Undergoing home hemodialysis

- On Continuous Ambulatory Peritoneal Dialysis (CAPD)

- On Continuous Cycling Peritoneal Dialysis (CCPD)

- Transplant recipients

- Diagnosed with diabetes

Delays in getting the proper treatment needed for chronic kidney disease may lead to the following complications:

- Fatal levels of potassium or hyperkalemia. This condition can lead to dangerous, and possibly deadly, changes in the heart rhythm.

- Increased risk of peritonitis or inflammation of the membranes of the abdominal wall and organs. Peritonitis is a life-threatening emergency that needs prompt medical treatment.

- Anemia or decreased supply in red blood cells. Anemia can make a patient tired, weak, and short of breath.

- Heart disease, heart attack, congestive heart failure, and stroke

- High blood pressure which can cause further damage to the kidneys and negatively impact blood vessels, heart, and other organs in the body.

- Fluid buildup in the body that can cause problems with the heart and lungs.

According to Medscape, the most common cause of sudden death in patients with ESRD is hyperkalemia, which often follows missed dialysis or dietary indiscretion. The most common cause of death overall in the dialysis population is cardiovascular disease; cardiovascular mortality is 10-20 times higher in dialysis patients than in the general population.

## Kidney Patients Who Wear a Medical ID Have 62% Lower Risk of Renal Failure

In a study of 350 patients, primarily in CKD stages 2 through 5, those who wore a medical ID bracelet or necklace had a 62% lower risk of developing kidney failure, based on eGFR. Wearing a medical-alert bracelet or necklace was associated with a lower risk of developing kidney failure compared with usual care.

Wearing a medical ID can serve as a reminder to look after your health and make the right choices such as taking medication on time and sticking to proper diet.

## 6 Things to Engrave on Kidney Disease Medical ID

A custom engraved medical alert jewelry can hold precise information that is specific to the wearer's health condition. Here are some of the most important items to put on a chronic kidney disease or kidney failure medical ID:

- Name
- Medical information – including if you have other medical conditions such as diabetes or high blood pressure
- Stage of CKD or kidney function
- Transplant information
- Current list of medicines

- Contact person

Some patients have a long list of medications that may not fit on the engraved part of an ID. An emergency wallet card is recommended to use for listing down your medicines and other information or medical history."

## 9/9/19 *You're Bringing What?*

I have stayed overnight in the hospital three times in my life: once for a concussion, of which I don't remember anything (No surprise there.), and twice for the birth of each of my daughters, of which I only remember the actual births. I'm facing a six to thirteen day stay towards the end of the month… and I just don't know what to bring or why. While it's not a kidney related stay, as Chronic Kidney Disease patients we all know CKD patients may need to stay in the hospital, too, for transplants, kidney cancer, or other reasons.

I got a call from the surgeon's office today. They were able to explain what to bring on the day of surgery: *nothing*. It seems there are no lockers to hold valuables while you're in surgery. While I took a breath to contemplate life without my phone and/or iPad, it was explained that I would probably be sleeping until the next day, anyway. I didn't know that. Hmmm, maybe I'll just bring a book – a real book – for that first day… just in case I wake up. I can bring a paperback so I won't care if it's 'mislaid.' Or can I?

All right, enough guessing. Let's do some researching here. This is from MedicineNet:

1. "Documents and paperwork. Ideally, you should bring all the necessary paperwork in one folder, preferably the kind with a tie or snap closure to guarantee that important documents will not be lost. Don't forget insurance cards, a list of all the medications you are currently taking, and a list of telephone numbers of family and friends. If you have a written power of attorney or living will, always bring those along with you too.

2. A small amount of money for newspapers, vending machines, and such. Bringing credit cards or large amounts of cash is not recommended, since theft can occur in hospitals. It is also a good idea to leave all jewelry at home, it is one less thing to worry about losing or being stolen.

3. Clothing. You may want to bring comfortable pajamas or lounging clothes, if you'll be able to wear your own clothing. Bring a supply of loose-fitting underwear and comfortable socks …. A cardigan-style sweater or bed jacket can help ward off the chills. Make sure you have slippers to walk around in the hospital and one pair of regular shoes (in case you're allowed to walk outside, and you'll need them for the trip home anyway).

4. Eyeglasses, if you require them.

5. Writing paper and pen, for making notes or recording questions you want to ask your doctor

6. A prepaid phone card for calls from your room telephone.

7. Toiletries. You can bring your toothbrush, toothpaste, lotion, deodorant, soap, shampoo, a comb or hair brush, and other toiletries from home, but avoid perfumes and any highly scented products. Lip balm is also a good addition to your toiletries kit.

8. Something to occupy your time – Bring books or magazines to help pass the time….

9. Photos or small personal items. Many people enjoy having a couple of small framed photos or mementos from home to personalize their hospital space.

10. Finally, check the hospital's policy about electronic items before you pack your laptop, portable DVD player, MP-3 or CD player, or cell phone. In particular, cell phone use is forbidden in many hospitals since it may interfere with electronic patient monitoring equipment. Don't forget that high-end electronic items can also be targets for theft – if you are allowed to bring them, make sure that a relative or friend takes them home or that they can be safely stored when you're sleeping or not in your room."

Now, wait a minute. I get it that MedicineNet may be referring to the day *after* surgery. But, in my case, that means I prepare a bag and give it to my daughter to bring the next day. The staff at the surgeon's office did tell me the hospital will provide a toothbrush and toothpaste, but will they allow me to bring the BiPap that I use for sleep apnea or the mouth piece I sleep with to prevent my jaw from locking? Let's look again.

U.S. News has some of the same items on their list:

**"To recap, here are 11 items to pack in your hospital bag.**

- Loose, warm and comfortable clothing.
- Your own pillow.
- Your own toiletries.
- Flip-flops.
- Earplugs and earphones.
- Comfort flicks.
- Escapist books.

- Laundry lists: of your medications, doctors and family and friends.

- Pen and paper.

- Scents.

- Drugstore supplies."

They also make a really good point about bringing you own medications and toiletries so you're not being charged for them by the hospital. I would avoid the scents just because so many people are scent sensitive these days.

I was still a bit confused, so I went to my hospital's website. I learned that not only are cell phones permitted, but Wi-Fi is offered for free. Great. What more can I find out about what to pack, I wondered. My biggest desire was for Shiloh, my comfort dog, to be with me but I knew that wasn't going to happen.

I thought VeryWellHealth was more realistic about what to pack and I especially appreciated the warnings about electronics:

"You won't have a lot of space to store things, so try to fit everything you need into a standard roll-on bag. Be sure that is well labeled and is lockable as an extra layer of security.

Among the things you should include on your packing checklist:

- Personal medications, preferably in their original container so that the nurse can find them for you if you are unable to reach them

- A list of your current medications to add to your hospital chart, including names, dosages, and dosing schedule

- Comfortable pajamas (loose-fitting is best)

- A light robe for modesty, especially in a shared room

- Slippers with rubber soles (to prevent slipping)

- Plenty of socks and underwear

- Toothbrush, toothpaste, and deodorant

- Hairbrush or comb

- Soap, skin care products, and hair care products if you prefer your own (ideally travel size)

- Special needs products like tampons, sanitary pads, or denture cream

- Glasses (which may be easier than contacts if you think you'll be dozing a lot)

- Outfit to wear home (something loose is best, also make sure it won't rub on your incision)

- A cell phone charger for your cell phone

- Your laptop charger if you intend to bring one

- Earplugs if you are a light sleeper

- An eyemask if you are used to black-out curtains

- Entertainment such as books, a portable DVD player, puzzles, or magazines

- Earbuds or earphones for your P3 or DVD player

- Non-perishable snacks, especially if you have dietary concerns (such as diabetes or chronic medications that need to be taken with high-fat foods)"

One quick call to the hospital to see if they have any additions to make to these lists and I'm ready to pack. How about you?

## 9/16/19 re·ha·bil·i·ta·tion

What! As if staying in the hospital for six to thirteen days weren't enough, it turned out that I would be in a rehabilitation center for an additional six to eight weeks. Again, while this was for pancreatic cancer, many Chronic Kidney Disease patients who have had surgery may require a stay in such places, too. I look for new experiences, but not this kind.

Let's go to my favorite dictionary, the Merriam-Webster Dictionary for the definition of the word.

"a: to bring (someone or something) back to a normal, healthy condition after an illness, injury, drug problem, etc.

b: to teach (a criminal in prison) to live a normal and productive life

c: to bring (someone or something) back to a good condition"

I hope it's clear that it's the first definition we're dealing with today.

Forgive me for being dense, but I still didn't get how that's going to be done. So I searched for help and MedlinePlus, which is part of the U.S. National Library of Congress which, in turn, is part of the National Health Institutes, did just that.

### "What happens in a rehabilitation program?

When you get rehabilitation, you often have a team of different health care providers helping you. They will work with you to figure out your needs, goals, and treatment plan. The types of treatments that may be in a treatment plan include

- Assistive devices, which are tools, equipment, and products that help people with disabilities move and function

- Cognitive rehabilitation therapy to help you relearn or improve skills such as thinking, learning, memory, planning, and decision making

- Mental health counseling

- Music or art therapy to help you express your feelings, improve your thinking, and develop social connections

- Nutritional counseling

- Occupational therapy to help you with your daily activities

- Physical therapy to help your strength, mobility, and fitness

- Recreational therapy to improve your emotional well-being through arts and crafts, games, relaxation training, and animal-assisted therapy

- Speech-language therapy to help with speaking, understanding, reading, writing and swallowing

- Treatment for pain

- Vocational rehabilitation to help you build skills for going to school or working at a job

Depending on your needs, you may have rehabilitation in the providers' offices, a hospital, or an inpatient rehabilitation center. In some cases, a provider may come to your home. If you get care in your home, you will need to have family members or friends who can come and help with your rehabilitation."

Personally, I won't need some of these such as cognitive rehabilitation, speech-language therapy, and vocational rehabilitation. Brain and speaking aren't involved in pancreatic surgery and I'm retired. You may be in the same situation if you have rehabilitation or you may not. It's a list that's made unique for each patient. I've got to remind you here that I'm not a doctor; this is a lay person giving her opinion.

Hmmm, it seemed pretty clear that each type of surgery requires its own sort of rehabilitation. Now that we know what's involved, let's see who would be involved if you required rehabilitation after a surgery. WebMD offered a succinct, easy to understand answer.

"**Who Works With You**

Different experts help with different parts of your rehab. Some people who might be on your team:

**Physiatrist.** He's a doctor who specializes in rehab. He tailors a plan to your needs and oversees the program to make sure it's going well.

**Physical therapist.** He teaches you exercises to improve your strength and the range you have when you move your arm, leg, or whatever part of your body had the operation.

**Occupational therapist.** He helps you regain the skills you need for some basic activities in your everyday life. He might teach you how to cook meals, get dressed, shower or take a bath, and use the toilet. He'll also show you how to use gadgets that can help you care for yourself more easily, such as a dressing stick or elastic shoelaces. Some occupational therapists will visit your home to make sure it's safe and easy for you to get around.

**Dietitian.** He'll help you plan healthy meals. If your doctor has told you to avoid salt, sugar, or certain foods after your surgery, the dietitian can help you find other choices.

**Speech therapist.** He helps with skills like talking, swallowing, and memory. Speech therapy can be helpful after surgery that affects your brain.

**Nurses.** They care for you if you're staying for a few weeks or months in a rehab center. They may also come to your home to help track your recovery and help you with the transition to life back at home.

**Psychologist or counselor.** It's natural to feel stressed out or depressed after your surgery. A mental health professional can help you manage your worries and treat any depression.

It can take many months to recover from an operation, but be patient. A lot depends on your overall health and the kind of procedure you had. Work closely with your rehab team and follow their instructions. Your hard work will pay off."

Looking over the list, I won't need a speech therapist and neither would you if you have some kind of kidney related surgery. I'm not so sure about a psychologist or counselor, either. I'm sort of thinking that going through chemotherapy and radiation treatments without one, I won't need one after surgery. Then again, I've never had major surgery before and I've been told this is *major* major surgery. However, should I find myself in a position where my medical team and/or I feel I need counseling, I would not hesitate to ask for it… just as I've asked for help with the cancer.

Rehabilitation offers so much. I had no idea this was available until my surgeon told me about it. Nor did I know that Medicare will pay for it… sort of. This is from Medicare.

"You pay this for each benefit period:

- Days 1-60: $1,364 deductible.*

- Days 61-90: $341 coinsurance each day.

- Days 91 and beyond: $682 coinsurance per each 'lifetime reserve day' after day 90 for each benefit period (up to 60 days over your lifetime).

- Each day after the lifetime reserve days: all costs.

*You don't have to pay a deductible for care you get in the inpatient rehabilitation facility if you were already charged a deductible for care you got in a prior hospitalization within the same benefit period. This is because your benefit period starts on day one of your prior hospital stay, and that stay counts towards your deductible."

Excuse me while I go check my bank account.

## 9/23/19 *It's Like the Sahara in There*

I like my dentist, especially when he tells me something I didn't know. When I went to see him last time, I told him my chemo experience and how dry my mouth was. I thought they might be related. He patiently gave me the same information as the Mayo Clinic did.

"Dry mouth, or xerostomia (zeer-o-STOE-me-uh), refers to a condition in which the salivary glands in your mouth don't make enough saliva to keep your mouth wet. Dry mouth is often due to the side effect of certain medications or aging issues or as a result of radiation therapy for cancer. Less often, dry mouth may be caused by a condition that directly affects the salivary glands.

Saliva helps prevent tooth decay by neutralizing acids produced by bacteria, limiting bacterial growth and washing away food particles. Saliva also enhances your ability to taste and makes it easier to chew and swallow. In addition, enzymes in saliva aid in digestion.

Decreased saliva and dry mouth can range from being merely a nuisance to something that has a major impact on your general health and the health of your teeth and gums, as well as your appetite and enjoyment of food.

Treatment for dry mouth depends on the cause."

The joke's on me. I developed dry mouth *before* the radiation treatments began. At least my salivary glands weren't having any issues of their own. It seems we discussed xerostomia at the right time.

Wait a minute. Something is pulling on my memory. Something

about Chronic Kidney Disease and dry mouth. Of course, periodontics and CKD. The Journal Of Clinical Periodontology had just what I was trying to remember. By the way, this is a fascinating free online library by John Wiley, a publisher I remember well from when I worked as an educator.

"Periodontitis had significant direct effect, and indirect effect through diabetes, on the incidence of CKD. Awareness about systemic morbidities from periodontitis should be emphasized."

In other words, if you have CKD or diabetes, make certain your dentist knows so he or she can monitor you for the beginning of periodontic problems. Just as with any other medical issue, the sooner you start treatment, the better. I can attest to this since I caught my pancreatic cancer early, which gave me a much better chance of eradicating it from my body.

The treatment for dry mouth seems simple enough, as explained by Healthline (Thank you again for the two awards!).

"Dry mouth is usually a temporary and treatable condition. In most cases, you can prevent and relieve symptoms of dry mouth by doing one or more of the following:

- sipping water often

- sucking on ice cubes

- avoiding alcohol, caffeine, and tobacco

- limiting your salt and sugar intake

- using a humidifier in your bedroom when you sleep

- taking over-the-counter saliva substituteschewing sugarless gum or sucking on sugarless hard candy

- over- the-counter toothpastes, rinses, and mints

If your dry mouth is caused by an underlying health condition, you may require additional treatment. Ask your doctor for more information about your specific condition, treatment options, and long-term outlook."

The sugarless gum works well for me and, as an added benefit, quelled the nausea from the radiation treatments, too. While I don't drink or smoke, I will have an occasional half cup of coffee when I can tolerate it. I didn't know this was something to be avoided. As both a CKD patient and a type 2 diabetic (Thanks, pancreatic cancer.), I was already avoiding salt and sugar. So, without realizing it, I was already helping myself deal with dry mouth. Lucky me.

That got me to thinking. What other problems could dry mouth cause? I went to NHS Inform to look for an answer. Indeed, this is a Scottish website, but a mouth is a mouth no matter where it's located, right?

- "a burning sensation or soreness in your mouth

- dry lips

- bad breath (halitosis)

- a decreased or altered sense of taste

- recurrent mouth infections, such as oral thrush

- tooth decay and gum disease

- difficulty speaking, eating or swallowing"

On a personal note, I found the halitosis embarrassing and the altered sense of taste frustrating. And here I'd been blaming the chemo for that. Maybe it was the chemo, although my age could also be the cause of my dry mouth. I do admit that 72 could be considered "aging."

My husband orders the groceries and we now have a pantry full of food I used to love but all taste, well, funny now. Poor guy, he was just trying to get me to eat when he ordered the food. He knew calorie intake is important when you're dealing with cancer.

I wondered what the symptoms of dry mouth were... well, other than a dry mouth, that is.

"Common symptoms include:

- A sticky, dry feeling in the mouth

- Frequent thirst

- Sores in the mouth; sores or split skin at the corners of the mouth; cracked lips

- A dry feeling in the throat

- A burning or tingling sensation in the mouth and especially on the tongue

- A dry, red, raw tongue

- Problems speaking or trouble tasting, chewing, and swallowing

- Hoarseness, dry nasal passages, sore throat

- Bad breath"

Thank you to WebMD for the above information.

Will you look at that! Just as diabetes can cause CKD and CKD can cause diabetes, bad breath (halitosis), soreness or burning sensation in the mouth can both be symptoms of dry mouth and problems caused by dry mouth.

Let's see now. What else can I tell you about dry mouth? DentistryIQ is a new site for me. They describe themselves as "… a leading source of information that helps dental professionals achieve excellence in their positions, whether that position is dentist, dental practice owner, dental hygienist, dental office manager, dental assistant, or dental school student." I went there to find out just how many people suffer from dry mouth.

"It is estimated to affect millions of people in the United States, particularly women and the elderly…. Current research indicates that approximately one in four adults suffer from dry mouth, and this figure increases to 40 percent in populations over the age of 55…."

This was back in 2006, and unfortunately are the most current figures I could find. Let us know if you find more current ones.

## 9/30/19 *Needling Me*

Years ago, as a young woman in my twenties (Could that really be at least 50 years ago????), I was horrified to discover I needed surgery for bleeding hemorrhoids. It was embarrassing, my younger self thought. It was private, my younger self thought. So my younger self looked for an alternative and discovered acupuncture. Not only would I be spared someone – even though that someone would be a doctor – dealing with private parts of my body, but I would also be spared the insult to the body that surgery can be... and my insurance covered it.

Hmmm, I was fully clothed and the needles didn't hurt although I had expected the process to be painful. Best? I did get relief from the bleeding hemorrhoids and avoided the surgery.

Remembering that incident today for some unknown reason, I wondered what – if anything – acupuncture could do for those of us with Chronic Kidney Disease. So, I went searching for information. But wait, I'm getting ahead of myself – as usual. Let's go back to talking about what acupuncture is.

"Acupuncture is a form of medical treatment that's been used for hundreds — even thousands — of years. Acupuncture originated in Asian medical practices. That's why many licensure and oversight boards use the term 'Oriental Medicine' to classify acupuncture.

Acupuncture is practiced by tens of thousands of licensed acupuncturists. Expert acupuncturists train for three to four years. The training includes both instruction in the use of needles and instruction in diagnosing conditions. Practitioners have direct supervision from another senior or expert practitioner.

In addition to this training, acupuncturists must undergo testing from a national board of examiners and continue to take instructional courses each year to maintain their license.

The American Medical Association accepts acupuncture as a medical treatment, and some insurance companies may cover the cost of treatment."

Thank you, Healthline for the above information.

The University of California, San Diego, School of Medicine, Center for Integrative Medicine in the Department of Family Medicine and Public Health had a succinct description of the process.

"First, your acupuncturist will ask about your health history. Then, he or she will examine your tongue's shape, color, and coating, feel your pulse, and possibly perform some additional physical examinations depending on your individual health needs. Using these unique assessment tools, the acupuncturist will be able to recommend a proper treatment plan to address your particular condition. To begin the acupuncture treatment, you lay comfortably on a treatment table while precise acupoints are stimulated on various areas of your body. Most people feel no or minimal discomfort as the fine needles are gently placed. The needles are usually retained between five and 30 minutes. During and after treatments, people report that they feel very relaxed."

PubMed, part of the US National Library of Medicine, National Institutes of Health concluded via a small, fairly recent study:

"Acupuncture at bilateral Hegu, Zusanli, and Taixi for 12 weeks reduced creatinine levels and increased eGFR levels. The study only provided a feasibility method for the treatment of patients with CKD. However, the results of this preliminary study warrant further investigation."

I think we all need a little help here to understand this conclusion. The three words we are not familiar with are all acupuncture points. The Acupuncture Massage College's site explained in language I could understand.

**"Large Intestine Channel: LI4, Hegu**
This point is located on the back side of the hand between the thumb and first finger. The primary use of this point is to relieve pain and treat inflammatory and feverish diseases.

**Stomach Channel: ST36, Zusanli**
This point is located on the front of the leg, just below the knee. It is helpful for digestive disorders. Research shows that using this point results in positive effects in treating anemia, immune deficiency, fatigue, and numerous diseases.

**Kidney Channel: KI3, Taixi**
This point is located just behind the inner ankle. It is used for disorders in several areas of the body, including sore throat, toothache, deafness, tinnitus, dizziness, asthma, thirst, insomnia, lower back pain and menstrual irregularities."

Inflammatory? CKD. Anemia? CKD. Immune deficiencies? CKD. Kidney? CKD? Now we know why acupuncture can help us. There seems to be a split among doctors as to whether it will or not, so you'll have to be careful to talk to your nephrologist. Some will give you an emphatic, "YES!" Others will give you a questioning look. And still others will ask you, "Why bother?" Be prepared with your answers. You don't want to alienate the doctor in charge of your treatment and you want to keep the lines of communication open. Well, at least I do.

If you're excited about the idea of acupuncture, you may be asking yourself how to find a good, safe practitioner. Sure you can look in the phone book, but – just as with any doctor – what would you know about how this particular acupuncturist functions? Before I had CKD, when I was plagued by another medical problem but had already moved to Arizona away from my NYC acupuncturist, I asked my stepdaughter about the acupuncturist she saw. If your nephrologist is onboard, you can ask for a referral. Sometimes, your primary care physician can be a good source here, too.

If you're not excited about acupuncture, don't push yourself. My husband tried it once to please me and swore never to do that again because he just didn't like it. Okay, he has other ways of dealing with his back pain. While I am in favor of acupuncture and plan to incorporate this into my medical team once I'm done with surgery and rehab, I also like peace in the house.

## 10/07/19 *Dapagliflozin/SGLT2 inhibitors*

I've been reading a lot about dapagliflozin lately. That's a word I didn't know. And this is the perfect opportunity to learn about it. Ready? Let's start.

The obvious first stop to my way of thinking was Medline Plus, part of the U.S. Library of Medicine, which in turn, is part of the Institutes of National Health.

"Dapagliflozin is used along with diet and exercise, and sometimes with other medications, to lower blood sugar levels in patients with type 2 diabetes (condition in which blood sugar is too high because the body does not produce or use insulin normally). Dapagliflozin is in a class of medications called sodium-glucose cotransporter 2 (SGLT2) inhibitors. It lowers blood sugar by causing the kidneys to get rid of more glucose in the urine. Dapagliflozin is not used to treat type 1 diabetes (condition in which the body does not produce insulin and, therefore, cannot control the amount of sugar in the blood) or diabetic ketoacidosis (a serious condition that may develop if high blood sugar is not treated).

Over time, people who have diabetes and high blood sugar can develop serious or life-threatening complications, including heart disease, stroke, kidney problems, nerve damage, and eye problems. Taking dapagliflozin, making lifestyle changes (e.g., diet, exercise, quitting smoking), and regularly checking your blood sugar may help to manage your diabetes and improve your health. This therapy may also decrease your chances of having a heart attack, stroke, or other diabetes-related complications such as kidney failure, nerve damage (numb, cold legs or feet; decreased sexual ability in men and women), eye problems, including changes or loss of vision, or gum disease. Your doctor and other healthcare providers will talk to you about the best way to manage your diabetes."

SGLT2 inhibitors? Hey, that was going to be next week's blog... or so ignorant me thought. The Food and Drug Administration (FDA) explains what a SGLT2 inhibitor is.

"SGLT2 inhibitors are a class of prescription medicines that are FDA-approved for use with diet and exercise to lower blood sugar in adults with type 2 diabetes. Medicines in the SGLT2 inhibitor class include canagliflozin, dapagliflozin, and empagliflozin. They are available as single-ingredient products and also in combination with other diabetes medicines such as metformin. SGLT2 inhibitors lower blood sugar by causing the kidneys to remove sugar from the body through the urine. The safety and efficacy of SGLT2 inhibitors have not been established in patients with type 1 diabetes, and FDA has not approved them for use in these patients."

There are also quite a few warnings about amputations and urinary tract infections caused by SGLT2 inhibitors on this site, although they are dated 8/20/18.

So it seems that dapagliflozin is one of several medications classified as SGLT2 inhibitor. So let's concentrate on SGLT2s inhibitors then. Hmmm, is this some medication requiring injections or do you just pop a pill? Pharmacy Times answered my question.

Wait a minute, dapagliflozin is not recommended if your GFR is below 60, or stage 3 CKD. Canagliflozin is not recommended if your GFR is below 45. Your kidney function is a big factor in whether or not this drug can be prescribed for you.

But why? Exactly how do the kidneys process this drug? Basically, the SLGT2 inhibitor prevents the glucose in your blood from reentering your blood stream after your blood has been filtered. The glucose has nowhere to go, so it exits your body via your urine along with the other wastes.

What about the side effects, since we already know the limitations of prescribing SLTG2 inhibitors? I thought WebMd might enlighten us and they certainly did.

"On Aug. 29, 2018, the FDA issued a warning that cases of a rare but serious infection of the genitals and area around the genitals have been reported with the class of type 2 diabetes medicines called SGLT2 inhibitors. This serious rare infection, called necrotizing fasciitis of the perineum, is also referred to as Fournier's gangrene.

SGLT2 inhibitors are FDA-approved for use with diet and exercise to lower blood sugar in adults with type 2 diabetes. SGLT2 inhibitors lower blood sugar by causing the kidneys to remove sugar from the body through the urine. First approved in 2013, medicines in the SGLT2 inhibitor class include canagliflozin, dapagliflozin, empagliflozin, and ertugliflozin. In addition, empagliflozin is approved to lower the risk of death from heart attack and stroke in adults with type2 and heart disease. Untreated, type 2 diabetes can lead to serious problems, including blindness, nerve and kidney damage, and heart disease.

Seek medical attention immediately if you experience any symptoms of tenderness, redness, or swelling of the genitals or the area from the genitals back to the rectum, and have a fever above 100.4 F or a general feeling of being unwell. These symptoms can worsen quickly, so it is important to seek treatment right away.

On May 15, 2015, the FDA informed the public that SGLT2 inhibitors have been associated with increased risk of ketoacidosis in people with diabetes.

Common side effects

The most common side effect of SGLT2 inhibitors include:

- Genital yeast infections in men and women
- Urinary tract infections (UTIs)
- Increased urination
- Kidney problems
- Flu like symptoms
- Constipation
- Nasal congestion
- Urinary discomfort
- Back pain

Serious side effects of SGLT2 inhibitors include:

- Kidney failure
- Hyperkalemia (high levels of potassium in the blood)
- Hypotension (low blood pressure)
- Ketoacidosis
- Increased cholesterol levels

- Serious urinary tract infections

- Increased bladder cancer risk

- Serious allergic reactions

- Low blood glucose (hypoglycemia) when combined with insulin or drugs that increase insulin production

- Dehydration"

Whoa. It looks like there will have to be some serious discussions with your nephrologist before you agree to taking a SLGT2 inhibitor should he or she suggest it. Make sure you have your list of questions ready and someone to listen carefully and take notes.

## 10/14/19 *Get the Lead Out*

In case you haven't heard yet, my youngest and her husband are having a little boy at the end of the month. I've noticed that, as millennials, their generation shares what they already have instead of running out to buy new as my generation – the baby boomers – did. One thing that was shared with them was a 16 year old crib in ace condition.

I thought it was painted white and got nervous about lead in the paint until I did a little digging. Luckily, the anti-lead paint laws came into existence 41 years ago in 1978.

Then I started to wonder what sustained lead exposure could do to someone with Chronic Kidney Disease and turned to one of my favorite sites to find out. According to the National Kidney Foundation,

"Having too much lead in your body can affect all the organs in your body, including the kidneys. When it affects your kidneys, medical experts call it 'lead-related nephrotoxicity.' ('Nephro' refers to your kidneys, and 'toxicity' refers to poison.') Kidney damage from lead exposure is very uncommon in the United States. In fact, most experts believe that kidney damage from lead is rare nowadays, especially in the United States and Europe.

It's believed that lead exposure causes less than 1% of all cases of kidney failure. It is usually related to jobs where workers are exposed to very high levels of lead, such as stained glass artists, metal smelters, and people who work in battery factories or remodel old homes. The low levels of lead found in drinking water, house paint, dirt, dust, or toys rarely causes kidney damage.

But if it does happen, it is usually only after many years of lead exposure (5 to 30 years). Also, it is more likely to affect people who are already at risk for kidney disease, or those who already have kidney disease. In children, however, even mild exposure over many years can lead to health effects later in life, including kidney damage."

Let's say (Heaven forbid!) that you were among the "less than 1% of all cases of kidney failure" caused by lead exposure. How would you even know you had lead poisoning? The National Institute for Occupational Safety and Health (NIOSH), part of the Centers for Disease Control and Prevention (CDC) had an answer ready for us.

"Lead poisoning can happen if a person is exposed to very high levels of lead over a short period of time. When this happens, a person may feel:

- Abdominal pain
- Constipated
- Tired
- Headachy
- Irritable
- Loss of appetite
- Memory loss
- Pain or tingling in the hands and/or feet
- Weak

Because these symptoms may occur slowly or may be caused by other things, lead poisoning can be easily overlooked. Exposure to high levels of lead may cause anemia, weakness, and kidney and brain damage. Very high lead exposure can cause death.

Lead can cross the placental barrier, which means pregnant women who are exposed to lead also expose their unborn child. Lead can damage a developing baby's nervous system. Even low-level lead exposures in developing babies have been found to affect behavior and intelligence. Lead exposure can cause miscarriage, stillbirths, and infertility (in both men and women).

Generally, lead affects children more than it does adults. Children tend to show signs of severe lead toxicity at lower levels than adults. Lead poisoning has occurred in children whose parent(s) accidentally brought home lead dust on their clothing. Neurological effects and mental retardation have also occurred in children whose parent(s) may have job-related lead exposure…."

Did you catch the mention of kidney disease? Now what? How is lead poisoning treated? Let's see what another favorite site of mine, The Mayo Clinic has to say:

"The first step in treating lead poisoning is to remove the source of the contamination. If you can't remove lead from your environment, you might be able to reduce the likelihood that it will cause problems. For instance, sometimes it's better to seal in rather than remove old lead paint. Your local health department can recommend ways to identify and reduce lead in your home and community. For children and adults with relatively low lead levels, simply avoiding exposure to lead might be enough to reduce blood lead levels.

**Treating higher levels**

For more-severe cases, your doctor might recommend:

- **Chelation therapy.** In this treatment, a medication given by mouth binds with the lead so that it's excreted in urine. Chelation therapy might be recommended for children with a blood level of 45 mcg/dL or greater and adults with high blood levels of lead or symptoms of lead poisoning.

- **EDTA chelation therapy.** Doctors treat adults with lead levels greater than 45 mcg/dL of blood and children who can't tolerate the drug used in conventional chelation therapy most commonly with a chemical called calcium disodium ethylenediaminetetraacetic acid (EDTA). EDTA is given by injection."

Is that safe for your kidneys? Uh-oh, according to WebMD, it may not be.

"When chelation therapy is used the right way and for the right reason, it can be safe. The most common side effect is burning in the area where you get the IV. You might also experience fever, headache, and nausea or vomiting. Chelating drugs can bind to and remove some metals your body needs, like calcium, copper, and zinc. This can lead to a deficiency in these important substances. Some people who've had chelation therapy also have low calcium levels in the blood and kidney damage."

It looks like this is another case when you'll have to present the information to your nephrologist and see what he or she advises in your particular case. If it's a primary care doctor who is treating you for lead poisoning, be certain to tell him or her that you CKD.

10/21/19 *Sodium Bicarbonate, Anyone?*

I belong to a number of social media Chronic Kidney Disease support groups. Time and time again, I've seen questions about sodium bicarbonate use. I never quite understood the answers to members' questions about this. It's been years, folks. It's time for me to get us some answers.

My first question was, "What is it used for in conjunction with CKD?" Renal & Urology News had a current response to this. Actually, it's from last June 19$^{th}$.

"Sodium bicarbonate treatment of metabolic acidosis in patients with chronic kidney disease (CKD) improves renal outcomes and survival, researchers reported at the 56th European Renal Association-European Dialysis and Transplant Association Congress in Budapest, Hungary.

In a prospective open-label study, patients with CKD and metabolic acidosis who took sodium bicarbonate (SB) tablets were less likely to experience a doubling of serum creatinine (the study's primary end point), initiate renal replacement therapy (RRT), and death than those who received standard care (SC)."

It may be current but what does it mean? Let's start with metabolic acidosis. Medline Plus, part of the U.S. National Library of Medicine which, in turn, is part of the National Institutes of Health explains it this way:

"Metabolic acidosis is a condition in which there is too much acid in the body fluids."

But why is there "too much acid in the body fluid?"

I like the simply stated reason I found at Healthline, the same site that deemed **SlowItDownCKD** among the Best Six Kidney Disease Blogs for 2016 and 2017.

"When your body fluids contain too much acid, it's known as acidosis. Acidosis occurs when your kidneys and lungs can't keep your body's pH in balance. Many of the body's processes produce acid. Your lungs and kidneys can usually compensate for slight pH imbalances, but problems with these organs can lead to excess acid accumulating in your body."

In case you've forgotten, pH is the measure of how acid or alkaline your body is. So, it seems that when the kidneys (for one organ) don't function well, you may end up with acidosis. Did you know the kidneys played a part in preventing metabolic acidosis? I didn't.

I went to MedicalNewsToday in an attempt to find out if metabolic syndrome has any symptoms. By the way, AHA refers to the American Heart Association.

"According to the AHA, a doctor will often consider metabolic syndrome if a person has at least three of the following five symptoms:

1. Central, visceral, abdominal obesity, specifically, a waist size of more than 40 inches in men and more than 35 inches in women

2. Fasting blood glucose levels of 100 mg/dL or above

3. Blood pressure of 130/85 mm/Hg or above

4. Blood triglycerides levels of 150 mg/dL or higher

5. High-density lipoprotein (HDL) cholesterol levels of 40 mg/dL or less for men and 50 mg/dL or less for women

Having three or more of these factors signifies a higher risk of cardiovascular diseases, such as heart attack or stroke, and type 2 diabetes."

Well! Now we're not just talking kidney (and lung) involvement, but possibly the heart and diabetes involvement. Who knew?

Of course, we want to prevent this, but how can we do that?

"You can't always prevent metabolic acidosis, but there are things you can do to lessen the chance of it happening.

**Drink plenty of water** and non-alcoholic fluids. Your pee should be clear or pale yellow.

**Limit alcohol**. It can increase acid buildup. It can also dehydrate you.

**Manage your diabetes**, if you have it.

**Follow directions** when you take your medications."

Thank you to WebMD for the above information.

Let's say – hypothetically, of course – that you were one of the unlucky CKD patients to develop metabolic acidosis. How could you treat it?

I went directly to the National Kidney Foundation to find out. This is what they had to say:

"We all need bicarbonate (a form of carbon dioxide) in our blood. Low bicarbonate levels in the blood are a sign of metabolic acidosis. It is a base, the opposite of acid, and can balance acid. It keeps our blood from becoming too acidic. Healthy kidneys help keep your bicarbonate levels in balance. Low bicarbonate levels (less than 22 mmol/l) can also cause your kidney disease to get worse. A small group of studies have shown that treatment with sodium bicarbonate or sodium citrate pills can help keep kidney disease from getting worse. However, you should not take sodium bicarbonate or sodium citrate pills unless your healthcare provider recommends it."

I'm becoming a wee bit nervous now and I'd like to know when metabolic acidosis should start being treated if you, as a CKD (CKF) patient do develop it. Biomed reassured me a bit.

"Acid–base disorder is commonly observed in the course of CKF. Metabolic acidosis is noted in a majority of patients when GFR decreases to less than 20% to 25% of normal. The degree of acidosis approximately correlates with the severity of CKF and usually is more severe at a lower GFR…. Acidosis resulting from advanced renal insufficiency is called uremic acidosis. The level of GFR at which uremic acidosis develops varies depending on a multiplicity of factors. Endogenous acid production is an important factor, which in turn depends on the diet. Ingestion of vegetables and fruits results in net production of alkali, and therefore increased ingestion of these foods will tend to delay the appearance of metabolic acidosis in chronic renal failure. Diuretic therapy and hypokalemia, which tend to stimulate ammonia production, may delay the development of acidosis. The etiology of the renal disease also plays a role. In predominantly tubulointerstitial renal diseases, acidosis tends to develop earlier in the course of renal insufficiency than in predominantly glomerular diseases. In general, metabolic acidosis is rare when the GFR is greater than

25–20 ml/min (Oh et al. 2004)."

At least I understand why the sodium bicarbonate and I realize it's not for me… yet.

## 10/28/19 *Gee, That Smells Nice*

Decades ago, when I was a newlywed and still in college, we lived on East 90$^{th}$ Street in New York City. The neighborhood was old; the building was old. It was old enough to have *that* odor, the one New Yorkers are still arguing about. One group says it's dead rats in the walls; the other says it's feline urine that's built up over the years. It was pretty rank.

At that time, I was a wannabe hippie, so I did what all the wannabe hippies did. I lit incense. It was powerful and it smelled nice. Opening the windows wasn't a helpful option since this was a dumbbell shaped apartment and people had been throwing garbage out the windows and down into the little airspace the shape of the apartment created for over a hundred years.

They'd been throwing it out the back windows, too. Nobody wanted to walk their garbage down the five flights from where I lived. What about the front windows, you ask. If you didn't mind car exhaust smoke or the shrill cries of children playing in the street, that would have been okay. I liked the sound of the children, but it didn't help me study.

We finally figured out this was not the best place for us to live, so we moved to an apartment in Forest Hills, a neighborhood in Queens. It smelled nice there. Our three windows opened on to a courtyard belonging to the apartment building behind us. There were trees and bushes galore. But we still lit incense. By this time, my then husband was a wannabe hippie right along with me.

I moved a lot in those years: New Rochelle in Westchester, Park Slope in Brooklyn, and Stapleton Heights in Staten Island. In each new home, I lit incense more from habit than anything else.

Finally, I moved to Arizona and kept all ten windows in my home open throughout the fall, winter, and spring. But in the summer with its extreme heat, they had to be closed…. So what did I do? That's right; I burned incense. Never once did I consider this might be some sort of health hazard.

Now I have pancreatic cancer which I know is caused by the ATM gene (Stop laughing, please. That really is the name of the gene.) and, in my case, is hereditary But I also have Chronic Kidney Disease. I got to wondering if there's any connection between the incense burning and the fact that I have CKD. So, I decided to explore that possibility.

But first, let me tell those who may not know just what incense is. Dictionary.com has a nice, easy definition:

1. "an aromatic gum or other substance producing a sweet odor when burned, used in religious ceremonies, to enhance a mood, etc.

2. the perfume or smoke arising from such a substance when burned.

3. any pleasant perfume or fragrance."

I popped over to The National Center for Biotechnology Information (NCBI), which is part of the US National Library of Medicine, which in turn is part of the National Institutes of Health, which is connected to PubMed. Why? Because I remembered reading something about incense on this site.

I know, I know. I freely admit I have weird reading habits, but remember: I'm retired. I can indulge in anything that catches my fancy now… including reading weird, seemingly random articles.

Anyway, this is what I learned from this study of daily incense burning by Chinese CKD patients in Singapore.

"Our study provides epidemiological evidence that long-term exposure to domestic incense smoke may contribute to the risk of ESRD in the general populations. We acknowledge the lack of information on kidney function at baseline as a limitation in our study, and recommend that the findings be corroborated by future studies that can demonstrate the deterioration in kidney function with time in incense users. Given the worldwide prevalence of incense burning, our finding has substantial public health implications. We advocate implementing strategies to reduce exposure to the emissions from domestic incense and educating the public about the importance of improving ventilation with the use of incense."

This is no surprise if you're thinking logically, but then again, who thinks about incense? Although I'll bet you'll be doing a little bit more thinking about it now. There are some problems here, though.

1. I'm not Chinese.

2. I don't live in Singapore.

3. I don't burn incense on a daily basis.

Hmmm, let's see if I can find anything else. While not specific to CKD, Healthline did have concerns.

"Incense has been used for thousands of years with many benefits. However, studies are showing incense can possibly pose dangers to health.

Incense isn't officially deemed a major public health risk comparable to smoking tobacco. Correct use to minimize risks hasn't yet been explored. Neither has the extent of its dangers been explored, since studies thus far are limited.

Reducing or limiting incense use and your exposure to the smoke may help lower your risk. Opening windows during or after use is one way to reduce exposure.

Otherwise, you can explore alternatives to incense if you're concerned about the risks."

I intend to open the windows the next time I use incense to cover that darned chemo smell I'm still emitting. Consider opening the windows the next time you choose to use incense, if you do.

Time for a little gratitude here. You know I've been dealing with pancreatic cancer since last March. During this time period, I've been invited to present at a conference in Tokyo, participate in both a radio show and a newspaper article, and be a member of a think tank in New Jersey. To be honest, I hadn't realized how much physical energy I put into my CKD awareness outreach. While I had to answer, "Not this year. Please keep me in mind for next year," I am thankful for these opportunities.

11/4/19 *Zap!*

To my surprise, hair started growing back in unexpected places after I finished chemotherapy. One place was my face. My face! And quite a bit of it, more than a bearded person would have. At least, that's how it looked to me. I was surprised no one mentioned it to me, but supposed they were just glad I was still alive. I wasn't worried. I'd just use laser hair removal… or would I? I do have Chronic Kidney Disease.

What did that mean as far as the laser hair removal? I remembered from when I'd had it done on the mustache area about seventeen years ago that it doesn't work on white hair. No problem with this currently. This facial hair was growing in black and thick.

My goodness, you'd think I'd just be thankful to be alive at this point, too. But as is often attributed to Mr. Shakespeare, "Vanity, thy name is woman." (Actually, he wrote "Frailty, thy name is woman," but no one seems to remember that.) So, time to explore what CKD limits there are with laser hair removal.

Let's start at the beginning with what it is. WebMD explained it this way:

"Laser hair removal is one of the most commonly done cosmetic procedures in the U.S. It beams highly concentrated light into hair follicles. Pigment in the follicles absorb the light. That destroys the hair."

Just in case you need reminders,

"A hair follicle is a tunnel-shaped structure in the epidermis (outer layer) of the skin. Hair starts growing at the bottom of a hair follicle. The root of the hair is made up of protein cells and is nourished by blood from nearby blood vessels.

As more cells are created, the hair grows out of the skin and reaches the surface. Sebaceous glands near the hair follicles produce oil, which nourishes the hair and skin."

Thank you to Healthline for that information. Notice I specified hair follicles since there are other kinds of follicles.

What else might we need defined. Oh yes, pigment. I used the definition of pigmentation instead since it was less convoluted to my way of thinking. The 'ation' part just means the action or process of whatever we're discussing – in this case pigment. MedicineNet tells us it's:

"The coloring of the skin, hair, mucous membranes, and retina of the eye. Pigmentation is due to the deposition of the pigment melanin, which is produced by specialized cells called melanocytes."

Now, the limitations with CKD – if any. In the last 17 years, I've learned that not only wouldn't white hair respond to laser hair removal, but gray and blonde won't either. It will also be less effective on red hair. It all has to do with your melanin.

Whoa! This was unexpected. I not only did NOT find any research warning about CKD and laser hair removal, but found some that endorsed it. For instance, The National Center for Biotechnology Information (NCBI), which is part of the U.S. National Library of Medicine, which in turn is part of the National Institutes of Health, which is connected to PubMed.

"Laser hair reduction is a well-established modality for a wide range of medical indications. Laser hair reduction can be beneficial for hemodialysis patients who undergo repeated adhesive tape application and removal at their hemodialysis site during hemodialysis sessions. There is a paucity of published literature on efficacious laser hair removal treatments for hemodialysis patients. Herein, we present a case of a 50-year-old male (Fitzpatrick III) with end-stage renal disease on hemodialysis, who achieved successful laser hair reduction at his hemodialysis vascular access site with five sessions of a neodymium:yttrium-aluminium-garnet (Nd:YAG) laser (1064 nm) to improve his quality of life by reducing the hair burden at the adhesive tape site application. We recommend providing this safe and effective hair reduction treatment option for hemodialysis patients given the decreased quality of life associated with end stage renal disease and hemodialysis. J Drugs Dermatol. 2018; 17(7):794-795."

Let me translate the medicalese. This abstract means that using laser hair removal around the patient's access site for dialysis made his life easier (and less painful) since the tape wasn't sticking to his arm or body hair anymore. We all know how painful taking off adhesive anything can be if body hair is involved.

I have dug around in my computer for hours and hours. That's all I found about laser hair removal and Chronic Kidney Disease. That's the great thing about keeping an open mind; you find some unexpected information.

Side note: Are you aware of Mrs. Dash's seasonings for use instead of salt? It's come to the point where I can taste even a teeny bit of salt. After almost a decade of not using salt, I've lost my taste for it... but Mrs. Dash? How does lemon pepper seasoning sound to you? Or garlic and herb? There are about 28 different flavors of seasoning. They also make marinades which was news to me. I usually choose the less spicy seasonings, but they have some zingers that you spicy food loving CKD patients will probably enjoy more.

## 11/11/19 *HIV and CKD*

Every morning, although I don't have enough energy yet to create original posts, I peruse the Facebook Chronic Kidney Disease pages, Twitter, Instagram, and even LinkedIn for current information about CKD. I was surprised to see a post seeming to claim that Human Immunodeficiency Virus (HIV) can cause CKD. How had I never heard about this before?

As usual when I don't know or understand something, I decided to investigate. My first stop was The National Institutes of Health.

- "The kidneys are two fist-sized organs in the body that are located near the middle of the back on either side of the spine. The main job of the kidneys is to filter harmful waste and extra water from the blood. (We know that already.)

- Injury or disease, including HIV infection, can damage the kidneys and lead to kidney disease.

- High blood pressure and diabetes are the leading causes of kidney disease. In people with HIV, poorly controlled HIV infection and coinfection with the hepatitis C virus (HCV) also increase the risk of kidney disease.

- Some HIV medicines can affect the kidneys. Health care providers carefully consider the risk of kidney damage when recommending specific HIV medicines to include in an HIV regimen.

- Kidney disease can advance to kidney failure. The treatments for kidney failure are dialysis and a kidney transplant. Both treatments are used to treat kidney failure in people with HIV."

Well, I knew there was a possibility of Acute Kidney Injury (AKI) leading to CKD, but HIV? What's that? Oh, sorry, of course I'll explain what HIV is. Actually, it's not me doing the explaining, but the Center for Disease Control (CDC).

"HIV stands for human immunodeficiency virus. It is the virus that can lead to acquired immunodeficiency syndrome or AIDS if not treated. Unlike some other viruses, the human body can't get rid of HIV completely, even with treatment. So once you get HIV, you have it for life.

HIV attacks the body's immune system, specifically the CD4 cells (T cells), which help the immune system fight off infections. Untreated, HIV reduces the number of CD4 cells (T cells) in the body, making the person more likely to get other infections or infection-related cancers. Over time, HIV can destroy so many of these cells that the body can't fight off infections and disease. These opportunistic infections or cancers take advantage of a very weak immune system and signal that the person has AIDS, the last stage of HIV infection.

No effective cure currently exists, but with proper medical care, HIV can be controlled. The medicine used to treat HIV is called antiretroviral therapy or ART. If people with HIV take ART as prescribed, their viral load (amount of HIV in their blood) can become undetectable. If it stays undetectable, they can live long, healthy lives and have effectively no risk of transmitting HIV to an HIV-negative partner through sex. Before the introduction of ART in the mid-1990s, people with HIV could progress to AIDS in just a few years. Today, someone diagnosed with HIV and treated before the disease is far advanced can live nearly as long as someone who does not have HIV."

So, it's not only HIV itself that can cause CKD, but also the drugs used to treat HIV.

The National Kidney Foundation offers some ideas about how to avoid CKD if you have HIV:

"Many people with HIV do not get kidney disease or kidney failure. Talk to your health care provider about your chances of getting kidney disease. If you have HIV, you can lower your chances by:

- Checking your blood pressure as often as your doctor recommends and taking steps to keep it under control

- Taking all your HIV medications as prescribed

- Asking your doctor about HIV drugs that have a lower risk of causing kidney damage

- Controlling your blood sugar if you have diabetes

- Taking medicines to control your blood glucose, cholesterol, anemia, and blood pressure if your doctor orders them for you

- Asking your doctor to test you for kidney disease at least once each year if you:

    - Have a large amount of HIV in your blood

    - Have a low level of blood cells that help fight HIV (CD4 cells)

- o  Are African American, Hispanic American, Asian, Pacific Islander, or American Indian

- o  Have diabetes, high blood pressure, or hepatitis C"

It seems to me that avoiding CKD if you have HIV is almost the same as taking care of your CKD if you didn't have HIV, except for the specific HIV information.

I now understand why it's so important to take the hepatitis C vaccine. I turned to UpToDate for further information about hepatitis C and HIV.

"The consequences of hepatitis C virus (HCV) infection in HIV-infected patients are significant and include accelerated liver disease progression, high rates of end-stage liver disease, and shortened lifespan after hepatic decompensation, in particular among those with more advanced immunodeficiency …. In the era of potent antiretroviral therapy, end-stage liver disease remains a major cause of death among HIV-infected patients who are coinfected with HCV …."

Remember that drugs leave your body via either your liver or kidneys. If your kidneys are already compromised by HIV or the medications used to treat your HIV, you need a high functioning liver. If your liver is compromised by hepatitis C, you need high functioning kidneys. I was unable to determine just what high functioning meant as far as your kidneys or liver, so if you find out, let us know.

Please be as careful as possible to avoid HIV, and if you do have it, pay special attention to being treated for it. I'd like it if you were one of the people who is "diagnosed with HIV and treated before the disease is far advanced [so that you] can live nearly as long as someone who does not have HIV."

### 11/18/19 *Is it Blood Sugar or the Pancreas?*

We all know diabetes raises your risk of developing Chronic Kidney Disease. But why? What's the mechanism behind the fact? As far as I'm concerned, it's time to find out.

Let's start with diabetes. The National Institute of Diabetes and Digestive and Kidney Diseases (NIDDK), part of the National Institutes of Health (NIH), which in turn is part of The U.S. Department of Health and Human Services offers this explanation.

"Diabetes is a disease that occurs when your blood glucose, also called blood sugar, is too high. Blood glucose is your main source of energy and comes from the food you eat. Insulin, a hormone made by the pancreas, helps glucose from food get into your cells to be used for energy. Sometimes your body doesn't make enough—or any—insulin or doesn't use insulin well. Glucose then stays in your blood and doesn't reach your cells.

Over time, having too much glucose in your blood can cause health problems. Although diabetes has no cure, you can take steps to manage your diabetes and stay healthy.

Sometimes people call diabetes 'a touch of sugar' or 'borderline diabetes.'"

Having just had a tumor removed from my pancreas, I'm well aware that it produces insulin as well as digestive enzymes. Without a pancreas to produce insulin, you would need insulin injections several times a day.

I got what diabetes is, but how it causes CKD was still not clear.

Well, not until I read the following from The American Diabetes Association.

"When our bodies digest the protein we eat, the process creates waste products. In the kidneys, millions of tiny blood vessels (capillaries) with even tinier holes in them act as filters. As blood flows through the blood vessels, small molecules such as waste products squeeze through the holes. These waste products become part of the urine. Useful substances, such as protein and red blood cells, are too big to pass through the holes in the filter and stay in the blood.

Diabetes can damage this system. High levels of blood sugar make the kidneys filter too much blood. All this extra work is hard on the filters. After many years, they start to leak and useful protein is lost in the urine. Having small amounts of protein in the urine is called microalbuminuria.

When kidney disease is diagnosed early, during microalbuminuria, several treatments may keep kidney disease from getting worse. Having larger amounts of protein in the urine is called macroalbuminuria. When kidney disease is caught later during macroalbuminuria, end-stage renal disease, or ESRD, usually follows.

In time, the stress of overwork causes the kidneys to lose their filtering ability. Waste products then start to build up in the blood. Finally, the kidneys fail. This failure, ESRD, is very serious. A person with ESRD needs to have a kidney transplant or to have the blood filtered by machine (dialysis)."

Hmmm, now that we know what diabetes is and how it can cause CKD, maybe we need to look at ways to attempt to avoid diabetes.

- "**Losing weight and keeping it off.** Weight control is an important part of diabetes prevention. You may be able to prevent or delay diabetes by losing 5 to 10 percent of your current weight. For example, if you weigh 200 pounds, your goal would be to lose between 10 to 20 pounds. And once you lose the weight, it is important that you don't gain it back.

- **Following a healthy eating plan.** It is important to reduce the amount of calories you eat and drink each day, so you can lose weight and keep it off. To do that, your diet should include smaller portions and less fat and sugar. You should also eat a variety of foods from each food group, including plenty of whole grains, fruits, and vegetables. It's also a good idea to limit red meat, and avoid processed meats.

- **Get regular exercise.** Exercise has many health benefits, including helping you to lose weight and lower your blood sugar levels. These both lower your risk of type 2 diabetes. Try to get at least 30 minutes of physical activity 5 days a week. If you have not been active, talk with your health care professional to figure out which types of exercise are best for you. You can start slowly and work up to your goal.

- **Don't smoke.** Smoking can contribute to insulin resistance, which can lead to type 2 diabetes. If you already smoke, try to quit.

- **Talk to your health care provider** to see whether there is anything else you can do to delay or to prevent type 2 diabetes. If you are at high risk, your provider may suggest that you take one of a few types of diabetes medicines."

This is a list from NIH: National Institute of Diabetes and Digestive and Kidney Diseases posted on MedLinePlus. Notice it's mentioned that this is for type 2 diabetes.

There are 11 different kinds of diabetes. Types 1 and 2 are the most common. WebMD explains what type 1 and 2 are.

"Type 1 diabetes is an autoimmune condition. It's caused by the body attacking its own pancreas with antibodies. In people with type 1 diabetes, the damaged pancreas doesn't make insulin…. With Type 2 diabetes, the pancreas usually produces some insulin. But either the amount produced is not enough for the body's needs, or the body's cells are resistant to it. Insulin resistance, or lack of sensitivity to insulin, happens primarily in fat, liver, and muscle cells."

This is all starting to make sense.

## 11/25/19 *Another Kind of Kidney Disease*

While I'm still recuperating, I've had plenty of time to read Twitter articles, among other things. One topic I've been reading about is lupus nephritis. I think we've all heard of lupus, but just in case, here's a definition from MedicineNet.

"A chronic inflammatory disease that is caused by autoimmunity. Patients with lupus have in their blood unusual antibodies that are targeted against their own body tissues. Lupus can cause disease of the skin, heart, lungs, kidneys, joints, and nervous system."

Did you catch the mention of kidneys in the above definition? That's where the nephritis part of the condition comes in. By now, we're all probably tired of being reminded that 'neph' means relating to the kidneys (although in non-medical terms, it means relating to the clouds) and 'itis' means inflammation. Nuts! I just reminded you again. Let's ignore that. So, lupus nephritis actually means

"… a kidney disorder [which] is a complication of systemic lupus erythematosus."

Thank you to MedlinePlus for the definition. Oh, "systemic lupus erythematosus" refers back to autoimmune disease. Still, the word "erythematosus" puzzled me. I finally figured it out after realizing I probably wasn't going to get a definition since almost all the entries were for lupus erythematosus. Remember, I studied Greek & Latin roots way, way back in college. It means red and is from the Greek. I get it. Sometimes, lupus patients have a red rash in butterfly form across their face.

So, how do you develop this particular kidney disease? What better place to find out than Lupus.org.

"Inflammation of the nephrons, the structures within the kidneys that filter the blood, is called glomerulonephritis, or nephritis. Lupus nephritis is the term used when lupus causes inflammation in your kidneys, making them unable to properly remove waste from your blood or control the amount of fluids in your body."

Hmmm, no lupus equals no lupus nephritis. However, if you do have lupus, you may develop lupus nephritis.

Let's say hypothetically that you or a loved one (or even your neighbor down the block) has lupus and is concerned about developing lupus nephritis. How would they know if they were developing it? I had to look no further than the National Kidney Foundation.

"Lupus nephritis can cause many signs and symptoms and may be different for everyone. Signs of lupus nephritis include:

- **Blood in the urine (hematuria):** Glomerular disease can cause your glomeruli to leak blood into your urine. Your urine may look pink or light brown from blood.

- **Protein in the urine (proteinuria):** Glomerular disease can cause your glomeruli to leak protein into your urine. Your urine may be foamy because of the protein.

- **Edema**: Having extra fluid that your kidneys cannot remove that causes swelling in body parts like your legs, ankles, or around your eyes.

- **Weight gain:** due to the fluid your body is not able to get rid of.

- **High blood pressure**

I know these may also be the symptoms of Chronic Kidney Disease, but if you have lupus, then they may be symptoms of lupus nephritis. To make things even more complicated, there are five different kinds of lupus nephritis depending upon which part of the kidney is affected.

I was wondering about tests to diagnose lupus nephritis, like we have blood and urine tests to diagnose CKD. Healthline (Now do you see why I was so thrilled to receive their Best Kidney Blogs Award two years in a row?) cleared that up.

**Blood tests**

Your doctor will look for elevated levels of waste products, such as creatinine and urea. Normally, the kidneys filter out these products.

**24-hour urine collection**

This test measures the kidney's ability selectively to filter wastes. It determines how much protein appears in urine over 24 hours.

**Urine tests**

Urine tests measure kidney function. They identify levels of:

- protein
- red blood cells
- white blood cells

## Iothalamate clearance testing

This test uses a contrast dye to see if your kidneys are filtering properly.

Radioactive iothalamate is injected into your blood. Your doctor will then test how quickly it's excreted in your urine. They may also directly test how quickly it leaves your blood. This is considered to be the most accurate test of kidney filtration speed.

## Kidney biopsy

Biopsies are the most accurate and also most invasive way to diagnose kidney disease. Your doctor will insert a long needle through your abdomen and into your kidney. They'll take a sample of kidney tissue to be analyzed for signs of damage.

## Ultrasound

Ultrasounds use sound waves to create a detailed image of your kidney. Your doctor will look for anything abnormal in the size and shape of your kidney.

Yes, I know these are the same tests that are used to diagnose CKD, but if you have lupus, they also can diagnose lupus nephritis.

Okay, now the biggie: How do you treat it if you do have it? The MayoClinic had some sobering news for us:

"There's no cure for lupus nephritis. Treatment aims to:

- Reduce symptoms or make symptoms disappear (remission)
- Keep the disease from getting worse

- Maintain remission
- Avoid the need for dialysis or a kidney transplant

**Conservative treatments**

In general, doctors may recommend these treatments for people with kidney disease:

- **Diet changes.** Limiting the amount of protein and salt in your diet can improve kidney function.

- **Blood pressure medications.** Drugs called angiotensin-converting enzyme (ACE) inhibitors and angiotensin II receptor blockers (ARBs) can help control blood pressure. These drugs also prevent protein from leaking from the kidneys into the urine. Drugs called diuretics can help you get rid of excess fluid.

However, conservative treatment alone isn't effective for lupus nephritis.

**Immune suppressants**

For severe lupus nephritis, you might take drugs that slow or stop the immune system from attacking healthy cells, such as:

- Steroids, such as prednisone
- Cyclosporine
- Tacrolimus
- Cyclophosphamide
- Azathioprine (Imuran)

- Mycophenolate (CellCept)
- Rituximab (Rituxan)

When immunosuppressive therapies don't lead to remission, clinical trials may be available for new therapies.

**Treatment options for kidney failure**

For people who progress to kidney failure, treatment options include:

- **Dialysis.** Dialysis helps remove fluid and waste from the body, maintain the right balance of minerals in the blood, and manage blood pressure by filtering your blood through a machine.
- **Kidney transplant.** You may need a new kidney from a donor if your kidneys can no longer function."

Help! Running out of room (but we're done for today anyway).

## 12/2/19 *Nephritis without the Lupus*

Recently, I wrote about Lupus Nephritis. As one reader pointed out, it is possible to have Nephritis without Lupus. Let's take a look at how that works.

According to MedicalNewsToday,

"Nephritis is a condition in which the nephrons, the functional units of the kidneys, become inflamed. This inflammation, which is also known as glomerulonephritis, can adversely affect kidney function.

The kidneys are bean-shaped organs that filter the blood circulating the body to remove excess water and waste products from it.

There are many types of nephritis with a range of causes. While some types occur suddenly, others develop as part of a chronic condition and require ongoing management."

Of course! 'Itis' means inflammation, while 'neph' means kidney. It's amazing what you can remember learning in college over 50 years ago when you're 72.

Hmmm, what do they mean by "many types of nephritis"? DoctorsHealthPress lists them for us:

"1. **Interstitial Nephritis**

Interstitial nephritis is characterized by swelling between the tubules and kidneys. The kidney tubules reabsorb water and important substances from kidney filtration, and substances are secreted through urination.

Interstitial nephritis can be acute or chronic in nature. Acute interstitial nephritis is typically the result of an allergic reaction. Over 100 different medications cause interstitial nephritis, such as antibiotics, non-steroidal anti-inflammatory drugs (NSAIDs), and proton pump inhibitors.

Non-allergic interstitial nephritis causes include high calcium levels, low potassium levels, and autoimmune disorders.

2. **Pyelonephritis**

Acute pyelonephritis is a severe and sudden kidney infection. Consequently, the kidneys will swell, which may lead to permanent damage. Frequent occurrences are known as chronic pyelonephritis.

The infection will begin in the lower urinary tract in the form of a urinary tract infection (UTI). Bacteria enter the body through the urethra and spread to the bladder. At that point, bacteria will travel from the ureters to the kidneys.

3. **Glomerulonephritis**

Glomerulonephritis refers to a range of kidney conditions that cause inflammation in the very small blood vessels in the kidneys, which are called glomeruli.

It is also called glomerular disease or glomerular nephritis. When the glomeruli become damaged, the kidney can no longer efficiently remove excess fluids and waste.

4. **Lupus Nephritis** [Gail here: This is the type I recently wrote about.]

Lupus nephritis is inflammation of kidneys caused by the autoimmune disease known as systemic lupus erythematous (SLE)—also called lupus. This is where the body's immune system targets its own tissues.

As many as 60% of lupus patients will later get lupus nephritis. The most common symptoms include dark urine, weight gain, high blood pressure, foamy urine, and the need for nighttime urination.

### 5. IgA Nephropathy (Berger's Disease)

IgA (immunoglobulin A) nephropathy is also called Berger's disease. The kidney disease occurs when the antibody IgA lodges within the kidneys.

Over time, this leads to local inflammation, which interferes in the kidneys' ability to filter waste from the blood. It is a progressive disease that may lead to end-stage kidney failure.

### 6. Alport Syndrome

Alport syndrome is an inherited disease caused by genetic mutations to the protein collagen. It can lead to kidney failure, hearing problems, and vision issues.

It will often run in families, and the severity is greater in men. Common symptoms include high blood pressure, protein in the urine, blood in the urine, and swelling in the ankle, legs, feet, and around the eyes.

The genetic types of Alport syndrome include X-linked Alport syndrome (XLAS), autosomal recessive Alport syndrome (ARAS), and autosomal dominant Alport syndrome (ADAS)."

I usually move on to symptoms next but – as you can see – DoctorsHealthPress already took care of that for us. Thank you to DoctorsHealthPress.

Healthline (Yep, that's the same Healthline that awarded SlowItDownCKD a place among the top six kidney disease blogs in both 2016 & 2017.) offered more detail about the cause of several acute nephritis diseases:

"**Interstitial nephritis**

In interstitial nephritis, the spaces between the kidney tubules become inflamed. This inflammation causes the kidneys to swell.

**Pyelonephritis**

Pyelonephritis is an inflammation of the kidney, usually due to a bacterial infection. In the majority of cases, the infection starts within the bladder and then migrates up the ureters and into the kidneys. Ureters are two tubes that transport urine from each kidney to the bladder.

**Glomerulonephritis**

This type of acute nephritis produces inflammation in the glomeruli. There are millions of capillaries within each kidney. Glomeruli are the tiny clusters of capillaries that transport blood and behave as filtering units. Damaged and inflamed glomeruli may not filter the blood properly….

**What causes acute nephritis?**

Each type of acute nephritis has its own causes.

**Interstitial nephritis**

This type often results from an allergic reaction to a medication or antibiotic. An allergic reaction is the body's immediate response to a foreign substance. Your doctor may have prescribed the medicine to help you, but the body views it as a harmful substance. This makes the body attack itself, resulting in inflammation.

Low potassium in your blood is another cause of interstitial nephritis. Potassium helps regulate many functions in the body, including heartbeat and metabolism.

Taking medications for long periods of time may damage the tissues of the kidneys and lead to interstitial nephritis.

**Pyelonephritis**

The majority of pyelonephritis cases results from *E.coli* bacterial infections. This type of bacterium is primarily found in the large intestine and is excreted in your stool. The bacteria can travel up from the urethra to the bladder and kidneys, resulting in pyelonephritis.

Although bacterial infection is the leading cause of pyelonephritis, other possible causes include:

- urinary examinations that use a cystoscope, an instrument that looks inside the bladder

- surgery of the bladder, kidneys, or ureters

- the formation of kidney stones, rocklike formations consisting of minerals and other waste material

**Glomerulonephritis**

The main cause of this type of kidney infection is unknown. However, some conditions may encourage an infection, including:

- problems in the immune system
- a history of cancer
- an abscess that breaks and travels to your kidneys through your blood

It certainly looks like there's a lot more to nephritis than we'd thought.

## 12/16/19 *Now What?*

Wow! It's the last month of 2019 already. You may have noticed there was no blog post last week. That's because I was unexpectedly hospitalized with just my iPhone on me and poor internet at the hospital not once, but twice. But I'm back in the office now.

Today is Dana's turn to have his request filled. Although, I do wish the reader who graciously agreed to wait until after I'd recovered from major surgery to have her questions answered would contact me again. With so many people at my computer while I was hospitalized, her questions have been, er, mislaid.

Okay, Dana, back to you. Uh-oh, your messages have seemed to disappear, too. Well, I guess that's the last time I allow anyone to use my computer. I do apologize. Please resend your questions.

Mind you all, I am not a doctor. I'm just a writer who's taught research writing and been a Chronic Kidney Disease, stage 3 patient for 11 years. Anything I suggest – or that anyone else suggests, for that matter – should be checked with your nephrologist before you act on it.

Hmmm, we have to hold off on both questions. Now what? I know. Let's look at a rare kidney disease. Are you game?

Well, will you look at that? I've already blogged about some of them on this list by the American Kidney Fund. Use the topic drop down on the right side of the blog at **gailraegarwood.wordpress.com** if you're seeking info on one of them or let me know if you'd like information about one I haven't yet written about. Use comment on the blog so your request doesn't get lost.

- Alagille syndrome
- Alport syndrome
- Amyloidosis
- Cystinosis
- Fabry disease
- Focal segmental glomerulosclerosis (FSGS)
- Glomerulonephritis
- Goodpasture syndrome
- aHUS (atypical hemolytic uremic syndrome)
- Hemolytic uremic syndrome (HUS)
- Henoch-Schönlein purpura
- IgA nephropathy (Berger's disease)
- Interstitial nephritis
- Minimal change disease
- Nephrotic syndrome
- Thrombotic thrombocytopenic purpura (TTP)
- Granulomatosis with polyangiitis (GPA)

Minimal change disease? Whatever could that be? And why is it labeled in plain, laymen English rather than medical terms that we'd have to look up? Let's find out.

According to the National Kidney Fund,

"Many diseases can affect your kidney function by attacking and damaging the glomeruli, the tiny filtering units inside your kidney where blood is cleaned. The conditions that affect your glomeruli are called glomerular diseases. One of these conditions is *minimal change disease (*MCD). Minimal change disease is a disorder where there is damage to your glomeruli. The disease gets its name because the damage cannot be seen under a regular microscope. It can only be seen under a very powerful microscope called an *electron microscope.* Minimal change disease is the most common cause of nephrotic syndrome in children. It is also seen in adults with nephrotic syndrome, but is less common. Those with MCD experience the signs and symptoms of nephrotic syndrome much quicker than they would with other glomerular diseases."

This is so logical it makes me wonder why the rest of medicine isn't. I was referring to the part about the electron microscope. Let's slow down a bit and take a look at "nephrotic syndrome" to ensure we fully understand what this disease is about.

The Mayo Clinic tells us,

"Nephrotic syndrome is a kidney disorder that causes your body to excrete too much protein in your urine.

Nephrotic syndrome is usually caused by damage to the clusters of small blood vessels in your kidneys that filter waste and excess water from your blood. Nephrotic syndrome causes swelling (edema), particularly in your feet and ankles, and increases the risk of other health problems."

Got it? Okay, then back to minimal change disease. How, in heaven's name, do you get it? Hmmm, after surfing the internet for a while, it's become clear the medical community doesn't yet know the cause of minimal change disease, although the following may be involved:

"The cause is unknown, but the disease may occur after or be related to:

- Allergic reactions
- Use of NSAIDs
- Tumors
- Vaccinations (flu and pneumococcal, though rare)
- Viral infections"

Thank you MedlinePlus (part of the U.S. National Library of Medicine, which is part of the National Institutes of Health).

All right then, maybe we could move on to the symptoms. This is clearly one of those times I wish I could understand medicalese. The best I could figure out is that, while kidney function remains normal, minimal change disease leads you right into nephrotic syndrome. That is a conglomeration of symptoms, as explained by the well-respected Merck Manual Consumer Version:

"Early symptoms include

- Loss of appetite
- A general feeling of illness (malaise)

- Puffy eyelids and tissue swelling (edema) due to excess sodium and water retention

- Abdominal pain

- Frothy urine

The abdomen may be swollen because of a large accumulation of fluid in the abdominal cavity (ascites). Shortness of breath may develop because fluid accumulates in the space surrounding the lungs (pleural effusion). Other symptoms may include swelling of the labia in women and, in men, the scrotum. Most often, the fluid that causes tissue swelling is affected by gravity and therefore moves around. During the night, fluid accumulates in the upper parts of the body, such as the eyelids. During the day, when the person is sitting or standing, fluid accumulates in the lower parts of the body, such as the ankles. Swelling may hide the muscle wasting that is progressing at the same time.

In children, blood pressure is generally low, and blood pressure may fall when the child stands up (orthostatic or postural hypotension). Shock occasionally develops. Adults may have low, normal, or high blood pressure.

Urine production may decrease, and kidney failure (loss of most kidney function) may develop if the leakage of fluid from blood vessels into tissues depletes the liquid component of blood and the blood supply to the kidneys is diminished. Occasionally, kidney failure with low urine output occurs suddenly.

Nutritional deficiencies may result because nutrients are excreted in the urine. In children, growth may be stunted. Calcium may be lost from bones, and people may have a vitamin D deficiency, leading to osteoporosis. The hair and nails may become brittle, and some hair may fall out. Horizontal white lines may develop in fingernail beds for unknown reasons.

The membrane that lines the abdominal cavity and abdominal organs (peritoneum) may become inflamed and infected. Opportunistic infections—infections caused by normally harmless bacteria—are common. The higher likelihood of infection is thought to occur because the antibodies that normally combat infections are excreted in the urine or not produced in normal amounts. The tendency for blood clotting (thrombosis) increases, particularly inside the main veins draining blood from the kidneys. Less commonly, the blood may not clot when clotting is needed, generally leading to excessive bleeding. High blood pressure accompanied by complications affecting the heart and brain is most likely to occur in people who have diabetes or systemic lupus erythematosus."

So, while the name of the disease is written in plain language, it's clear this is a more complicated rare kidney disease than that would suggest.

12/23/19 *AKI & CKD*

Dana contacted me and here's the blog I promised him. (Still looking for the request from the woman who waited so patiently for me to recover from my surgery. Please contact me again.) Dana asked about AKI, Acute Kidney Injury, and how aggressively his nephrologist should be pursuing treatment of this. He and his nephrologist feel that his AKI may have been caused by strep.

I know I write about CKD, Chronic Kidney Disease, so what is AKI? The glossary in my very first CKD book, **What Is It and How Did I Get It? Early Stage Chronic Kidney Disease**, tells us 'acute' means:

"Extremely painful, severe or serious, quick onset, of short duration; the opposite of chronic."

This is what I wrote about AKI and CKD in **SlowItDownCKD 2017**,

"I'd always thought that AKI and CKD were separate issues and I'll bet you did, too. But Dr. L.S. Chawla and his co-writers based the following conclusion on the labor of epidemiologists and others. (Note: Dr. Chawla et al wrote a review article in the *New England Journal of Medicine* in 2014.)

'Chronic Kidney Disease is a risk factor for acute kidney injury, acute kidney injury is a risk factor for the development of Chronic Kidney Disease, and both acute kidney injury and Chronic Kidney Disease are risk factors for cardiovascular disease. Not surprisingly, the risk factors for AKI {Once again, that's acute kidney injury.} are the same as those for CKD… except for one peculiar circumstance. Having CKD itself can raise the risk of AKI 10 times.'

Whoa! If you're Black, of an advanced age {Hey!}, or have diabetes, you already know you're at risk for CKD, or are the one out of nine (Update: Now one out of seven.) in our country that has it. Once you've developed CKD, you've just raised the risk for AKI 10 times. I'm getting a little nervous here....

It makes sense, as researchers and doctors are beginning to see, that these are all connected. I'm not a doctor or a researcher, but I can understand that if you've had some kind of insult to your kidney, it would be more apt to develop CKD.

And the CVD risk? Let's think of it this way. You've had AKI. That period of weakness in the kidneys opens them up to CKD. We already know there's a connection between CKD and CVD (Cardiovascular Disease). Throw that AKI into the mix, and you have more of a chance to develop CVD whether or not you've had a problem in this area before. Let's not go off the deep end here. If you've had AKI, you just need to be monitored to see if CKD develops and avoid nephrotoxic {Kidney poisoning} medications such as NSAIDS… contrast dyes, and radioactive substances. This is just so circular!

As with CKD, your hypertension and diabetes {if you have them} need to be monitored, too. Then there's the renal diet, especially low sodium foods. The kicker here is that no one knows if this is helpful in avoiding CKD after an AKI… it's a 'just in case' kind of thing to help ward off any CKD and possible CVD from the CKD."

Dana's nephrologist put him on a regiment of prednisone for two months. Why? Well, prednisone is an anti-inflammatory drug. WebMD offers the following as possible causes of AKI. Notice the very last one and you'll see how prednisone may be helpful.

1. **"Something is stopping blood flow to your kidneys.** It could be because of:

- An infection

- Liver failure

- Medications (aspirin, ibuprofen, naproxen, or COX-2 inhibitors, like Celebrex)

- Blood pressure medications

- Heart failure

- Severe burns or dehydration

- Blood or fluid loss

2. **You have a condition that's blocking urine from leaving your kidneys. This could mean:**

- Bladder, cervical, colon or prostate cancer

- Blood clots in your urinary tract

- An enlarged prostate

- Kidney stones

- Nerve damage in your bladder

3. **Something has directly damaged your kidneys, like:**

- Blood clots

- Cholesterol deposits

- Medications that can directly damage kidneys, including NSAIDs like ibuprofen and naproxen, chemotherapy, and antibiotics

- Glomerulonephritis (inflamed kidney filters; can be caused by an infection, autoimmune disease (like lupus), multiple myeloma, scleroderma, chemotherapy drugs, antibiotics, or other toxins)"

Now we know AKI and Acute Kidney Failure are not the same thing, but it is possible that this nephrologist is using prednisone in an attempt to avoid Acute Kidney Failure?

One thing Dana asked that made me stop cold is "How do you cope with the inevitable aspects?" They are not inevitable, Dana. I am a lay person who has managed to keep my CKD at stage 3 for 11 years. I am also not a magician. What I am is someone who follows the guidelines for keeping my kidneys as healthy as possible.

You've already seen a nutritionist – hopefully a renal nutritionist, since a healthy diet is not necessarily a renal healthy diet – so you're aware of the nutrition aspect of protecting your kidneys. But there's more. Do you smoke or drink? If so, stop. Do you exercise? If not, start... but with your nephrologist's supervision. Are you getting adequate sleep and rest? Here's the hardest guideline: try to avoid stress. Of course, if you have a stressful life, avoiding stress can just be another stress.

As to how aggressively you should expect your nephrologist to treat your AKI (or the CKD resulting from it) really depends upon you and your nephrologist. For example, some think stage 3 is barely CKD and urge you to just keep watch. Others, like my nephrologist, take CKD seriously and have their nutritionists train you re the renal diet and speak with you themselves about the guidelines. As for AKI, again it depends on you, your nephrologist, and the severity of the AKI. Since you have waste product buildup and inflammation, you may need dialysis or a hospital stay... or watchful waiting while taking a medication such as prednisone.

There seems to be quite a lot of leeway as to the treatment you and your nephrologist decide upon.

## 12/30/19 *Auld Lang Syne Already?*

It's the last few days of 2019 and this year has whizzed by. My dance with pancreatic cancer has been a trip I could have done without, but the birth of my grandson more than made up for it. Now I get to see him all the time and I only have one more regiment of chemotherapy to go.

Oh, there I go again assuming everyone knows what Auld Lange Syne is. According to Classic FM:

**"What does 'Auld Lang Syne' mean?**

The most accurate plain English interpretation of the Auld Lang Syne's famous title is 'Old long since', or 'For the sake of old times'.

The song itself is reflective in nature, and is basically about two friends catching up over a drink or two, their friendship having been long and occasionally distant.

The words were written by Scottish poet Robert Burns in 1788, but Burns himself revealed at the time of composing it that he had collected the words after listening to the verse of an old man on his travels, claiming that his version of 'Auld Lang Syne' marked the first time it had been formally written down.

However, an earlier ballad by James Watson, named 'Old Long Syne', dates as far back as 1711, and use of the title phrase can be found in poems from as early as the 17th century, specifically works by Robert Ayton and Allan Ramsay."

The song is usually sung at the stroke of midnight on New Year's Eve and is closely associated with the ending of one year and the beginning of the next. That's tomorrow night.

Before we leave 2019, let's take a look at what's been happening in the kidney world this year.

The ball got rolling, so to speak, with this announcement:

"The Advancing American Kidney Health initiative, announced on July 10, 2019 by the US Department of Health and Human Services (HHS), places the kidney community in the national spotlight for the first time in decades and outlines a national strategy for kidney diseases for the first time …. In order to achieve the Advancing American Kidney Health initiative's lofty goals and make good on the KHI's commitment to people with kidney diseases, drug and device innovation needs to accelerate."

You can read the entire announcement from the Clinical Journal of the American Society of Nephrology.

The American Kidney Fund announced prizes for innovations in dialysis. We are now in phase two.

"HHS and ASN collaborated with patients, nephrologists, researchers and others in planning the competition. Several agencies, including the National Institutes of Health, the Food and Drug Administration, and the Centers for Medicare & Medicaid Services, are involved in this effort. AKF has provided comments to the KidneyX project, urging a focus on unmet needs and improving patient quality of life.

The KidneyX: Redesign Dialysis competition will have two phases. During phase one (late-October 2018-February 2019), innovators will be asked to come up with ideas to 'replicate normal kidney functions and improve patient quality of life.' During phase two

(April 2019-January 2020), innovators will be asked to develop prototypes to test their ideas."

You can also read my blog about KidneyX by using the topic dropdown on the right side of the blog at **gailraegarwood.wordpress.com**.

S.1676/H.R 3912 was passed this year, too. According to Renal Support Network, this is what the act provides:

"Specifically, the legislation does the following:

- Medigap available to all ESRD Medicare beneficiaries, regardless of age.

- Improve care coordination for people on dialysis by requiring hospitals to provide an individual's health and treatment information to their renal dialysis facility upon their discharge. The individual or dialysis facility may initiate the request.

- Increase awareness, expand preventative services, and improve coordination of the Medicare Kidney Disease Education program by allowing dialysis facilities to provide kidney disease education service. And it will allow physician assistants, nurse practitioners, and clinical nurse specialists, in addition to physicians, to refer patients to the program. And additionally, provide access to these services to Medicare beneficiaries with Stage 5 (CKD) not yet on dialysis.

- Incentivize innovation for cutting-edge new drugs, biologicals, devices, and other technologies by maintaining an economically stable dialysis infrastructure. The Secretary

- would be required to establish a process for identifying and determining appropriate payment amounts for incorporating new devices and technologies into the bundle.

- Improve the accuracy and transparency of ESRD Quality Programs so patients can make better decisions about their care providers.

- Improve patient understanding of palliative care usage as well as access to palliative care services in underserved areas.

- Allow individuals with kidney failure to retain access to private insurance plans as their primary payor for 42 months, allowing people to keep their private plans longer."

I scooted over to EurekAlert! when I realized they were announcing a drug I'd blogged about:

"'A drug like canagliflozin that improves both cardiovascular and renal outcomes has been eagerly sought by both patients with Type 2 diabetes and clinicians caring for them,' added Kenneth Mahaffey, MD, professor of medicine at the Stanford University School of Medicine and co-principal investigator of the trial. 'Now, patients with diabetes have a promising option to guard against one of the most severe risks of their condition.'

The researchers found the drug canagliflozin, a sodium glucose transporter 2 (SGLT2) inhibitor, was less effective at lowering blood sugar in people with reduced kidney function but still led to less kidney failure, heart failure and cardiovascular events such as heart attacks, strokes and death from cardiovascular disease.

Professor Perkovic said the results were impressive. 'The substantial benefit on kidney failure despite limited effects on blood glucose suggest that these drugs work in a number of different ways beyond their effects on blood sugar. This is an area of intense ongoing research.'"

These are just a few of the innovations in kidney disease in 2019. I hope to see many more for us – like the FDA approval of the artificial kidney – in 2020.

Until next year,

Keep living your life!

## Index

*1in9*, 41, 48, 52, 56, 61, 64

**A**

AAKP, See American Association of Kidney Patients.

Acupuncture, 179-82

Acute Kidney Injury, 206, 232-6, 260

AKI, See Acute Kidney Injury.

Albumin, 72-3, 82-3, 135, 211

Aldosterone, 79, 95-6

Alpha Lipoic Acid, 116-20

American Association of Kidney Patients, 133-4

American Kidney Health Initiative, 238

Anemia, 88, 92-3, 108-9, 160, 181, 190, 207

Antidote.com, 88-90

Anxiety, 23-7

Autoimmune Disease, 214, 222, 235

**B**

B12, See Vitamin B12.

Bartter Syndrome, 95-100

Biologic, 101-6

Biosimilar, 101-6

Blood Pressure Monitor, 21

Blood Pressure, 5-7, 10, 13, 41, 52-4, 72-3, 78, 83-4, 151-2, 160-1, 186, 193, 205, 207-8, 216, 218-9, 222, 230-1

Blood Transfusion, 91-4, 100,

Blood type, 94, 122-3

Bookmednow, 67-71

## C

Calcium, 35, 82, 95, 138-41, 191, 221, 230

Canagliflozin, 184, 240-1

Cancer, 29, 35-7, 91-2, 101, 111, 118-20, 126-30, 206, 225, 234

Clinical Trials, See Antidote.com and Clinicaltrials.com.

Clinicaltrials.com, 23, 86-90, 133-4

Creatinine, 74-5, 83, 139-40, 180-1, 192, 216

## D

Dapagliflozin, 183-7

DaVita Kidney Care, 42

Diabetes, 72-5, 111-3, 151-2, 175, 183-5, 194, 210-3, 240

Dialysis Travel, See Bookmednow.

Diet, 29, 53-4, 85, 124, 218, 233

Dragon Fruit, See Pitaya.

Dry Mouth, 174-8

## E

Edema, 132-3, 135-7, 215, 230

Erythropoietin, 92, 105

**F**

Facebook Support Groups, 61-2

Fiber, 28-34

Flu, See Influenza.

Focal Segmental Glomerulosclerosis, 81-5, 227

FSGS, See Focal Segmental Glomerulosclerosis.

**H**

Havimat, 132-3, 135, 137

HIV, See Human Immunodeficiency Virus.

Hospital Stay, 163-8

Human Immunodeficiency Virus, 205-9

**I**

Incense, 197-200

Influenza, 8-11

Infusion, 108-10

Innovations in Dialysis Prize Announcement, 238-9

International Society of

ISN, See International Society of Nephrology.

**K**

KDIGO, See Kidney Disease: Improving Global Outcomes.

Kidney Diet, See Diet.

Kidney Disease: Improving Global Outcomes, 22

KidneyX, 238-9

**L**

Laser Hair Removal, 201-3

Lead Poisoning, 188-91

Legislation (S. 1676/H.R. 3912), 239-40

Lind, James, 68

Lupus, 220-5

Lupus Nephritis, 214-9

Lymphedema, 133, 142-5

**M**

Medical Alert IDs, 159-62

Medications, 183-7, 218, 234

Metabolic Acidosis, 192-5

Metabolic Syndrome, 193-4

Minimal Change Disease, 227-9

Mrs. Dash's Spices, 203-4

**N**

Kidney Month, 40-3

Nephritis, 220-5

Neulasta, 101

Neuropathy, 111-20, 131-3, 135-7, 146-9

Nuclear Medicine Testing, 15-8

**O**

Occupational Therapy, 131-3, 135, 137, 146-9, 170-2

**P**

Pancreas, 35-9, 75, 112-3, 210-3

Parathyroid Hormone, 138-41

Pitaya, 20

Platelets, 91-4, 107-10, 122-3

Podcast, 63, 124

Potassium, 35, 76-80, 95-100, 160, 224

Protein, 37, 76, 84, 108, 123, 135-6, 143-5, 150-8, 211

Protein Buildup, 143-5

Proteinuria, 150-8, 215

**R**

Radiation, 118-20, 126-30

Red Blood Cells, 76, 91-3, 105, 107-8, 123, 160, 216

Rehabilitation Center, 169-73

Renal Diet, See Diet.

**S**

SGLT2 Inhibitors, 183-7

Sinusitis, 12-4

Sjögren's Syndrome, 76-80

Sodium Bicarbonate, 192-6

**T**

Tubules, 220, 223

**U**

Uromodulin Kidney Disease, 19-20

**V**

Vitamin B12, 116, 119-20

**W**

World Kidney Day, 44-7

**My Notes –**

## Have you read my previous Chronic Kidney Disease books?

## Available on Amazon.com and B&N.com

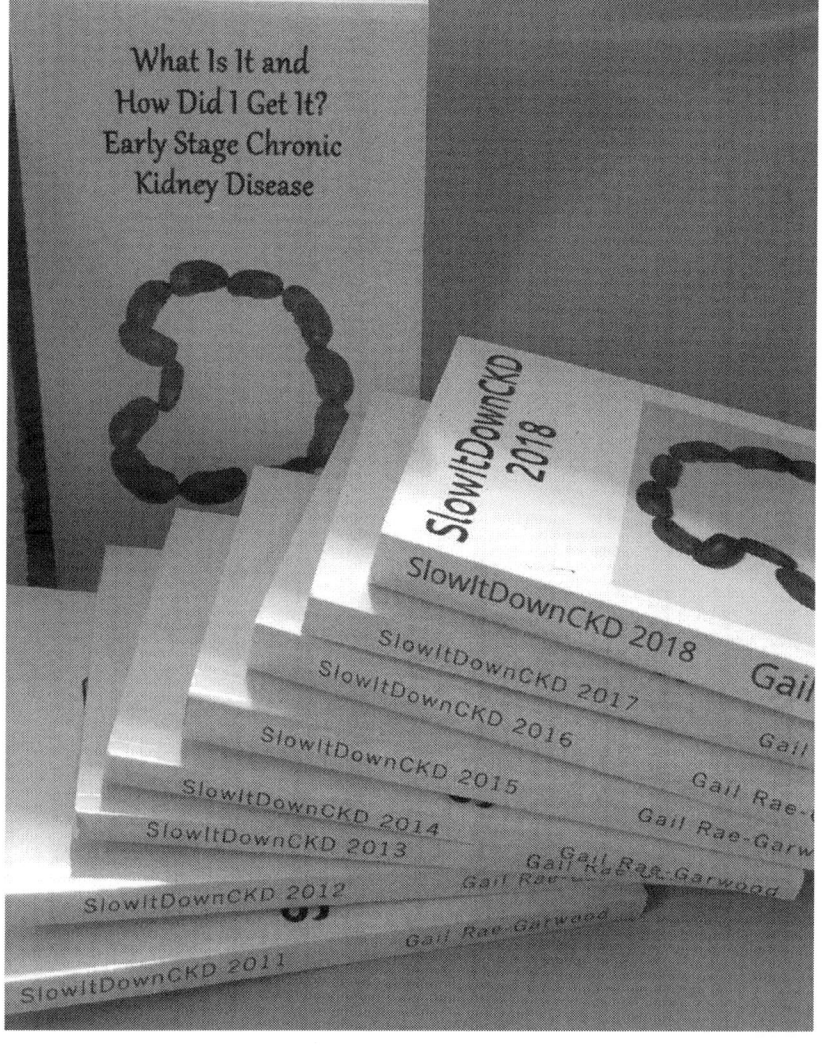

Follow the blog at **https://gailraegarwood.wordpress.com**

**SLOWITDOWNCKD**
EARLY AND MODERATE STAGE CHRONIC KIDNEY DISEASE

On Twitter, Pinterest, or Instagram, go to **@SlowItDownCKD**

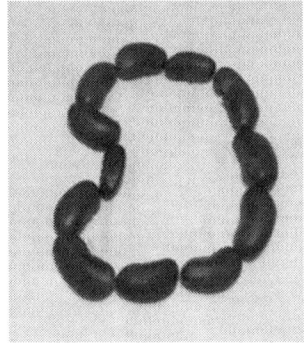

You can find me on LinkedIn as **Gail Rae-Garwood**

And then, there's the Facebook page at

*https://www.facebook.com/SlowItDownCKD/*

You can email me at **SlowItDownCKD@gmail.com**

And don't forget my website at **gail-raegarwood.com**

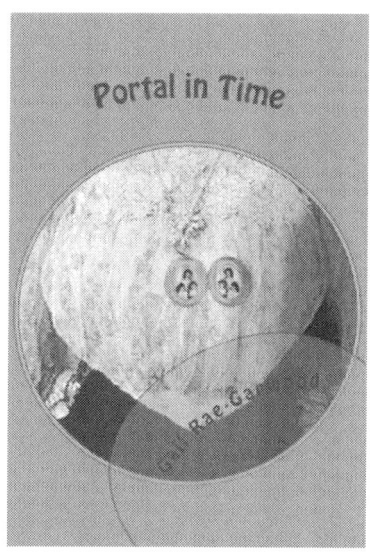

*If you'd like to read a time travel romance (above) or creative non-fiction based on others' experiences (below), I've written one of each. Both are available on Amazon.com and B&N.com.*

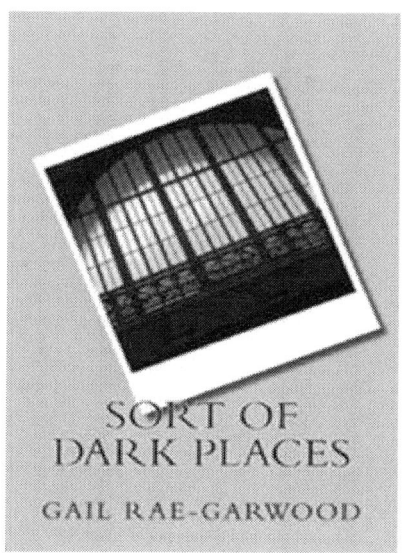

Printed in Great Britain
by Amazon